BRENDA BU

CANCER
QUIPS

Happy Reading!

Brenda Burling x

A collection of positive and uplifting tales shared by those who have experienced life with the BIG C

FOR EVERYONE

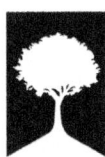

First Published in 2024
Matthew James Publishing
(an imprint of Andrews UK Limited)
West Wing Studios
Unit 166, The Mall
Luton, LU1 2TL

www.matthewjamespublishing.com

ISBN: 9781837914517

Text copyright © 2024 Brenda Burling
The moral rights of the author(s) have been asserted.

Apart from any fair dealing for the purpose of research, or private study, or criticism or review as permitted under the Copyright, Designs and Patents Act, 1988, this publication may only be reproduced, stored or transmitted in any form, or by any means, with the prior permission of the publisher, or in the case of reprographic reproduction, in accordance with the terms of licenses issued by the Copyright Licensing Agency. Enquiries concerning reproduction outside those terms should be sent to the publisher.

ONE EDITION, ONE AIM!

Provide support and positivity to all and smash taboos...
CANCER SUCKS!

Welcome to the compilation edition of *Might Make You Smile* and *Good For a Grin*, this is the most inclusive edition, ecologically friendly too with two books pulled in to one.

Both books were only ever going to be possible if people were prepared to do one thing...talk.

I was in luck! Finding the best places to connect with people who may actually consider sharing their cancer experiences was made so much easier by the amazing folk who have attended, supported and been involved with such organisations as the fabulous Brafternoon, Oddballs Foundation, Maggie's centres (in particular Maggie's Cambridge), Life Kitchen and particularly Ryan Riley directly. Word of mouth generated delightful connections and of course social media. Sadie Nine, BBC presenter, singer, actor and cancer survivor even came along to Brafternoon to share her stories personally, an afternoon of laugh out loud moments providing a massive supportive boost for all. Steve Harper former Newcastle United and Hull City goalkeeper shared his endorsement for *Good For a Grin*, particularly appropriate with so many contributors finding sport, rugby and football especially, a great positive component in their lives. All have been beyond generous with their time and input. The end result is what you see before you.

For the ladies we have smile inducing make-up disasters, wardrobe malfunctions and hairdressing hacks to name but a few.

For the gentlemen, some painful rugby match shenanigans, fertility clinic faux pas and mind blowing, honest, uplifting and informative blogging thanks to Dan Cook and Patrick Reeve.

Http://rugbysavedmylife.blogspot.co.uk (Dan Cook)
https://http2279.wordpress.com (Patrick Reeve)

HAPPY READING ALL!

Good For A Grin

RUGBY SAVED MY LIFE...

Or so my mate says.

Dan was a rugby man, which made his wife a rugby 'widow'. Unlike a football widow, she would wait for her beloved to come home to regale her with a blow-by-blow account (yes, in rugby terms this is a literal thing – black eyes and a variety of injuries always accompany the account and are always sported with a large degree of pride). Dan, however, was a rugby man with a sore testicle. The testicle in question had been giving him some grief. Dan was convinced it was just another of those 'rugby' injuries. Just how much it affected him, however, was brought home during a full 'hands on' incident in the middle of a match, which left him in absolute agony, having never felt such excruciating pain before.

As anyone who has the vaguest understanding of rugby will know, injuries are like trophies to all, bar the wives and girlfriends of rugby players. Getting your nuts bashed, along with every other part of your body, is nothing new. This is rugby after all, there's no crying over a broken nail here.

It was only when Dan (at the behest of his wife – yes, they really do know best) had a swollen gland in his neck checked out that he bit the bullet, manned up and said: "While I'm here, Doc, would you mind checking my testicles. I'm not sure everything is right." Dan was given the diagnosis he dreaded most, it was suspected he had testicular cancer. A referral to a consultant was agreed.

For a number of reasons, Dan decided to blog his experiences from the moment he was diagnosed. One, he could share his experiences with anyone else who might find themselves in the same situation, thereby giving himself the opportunity to look back and recollect how far he had come; and secondly, so his wife Nat didn't have to keep relaying the same information to people over and over again. He also wanted to document both the treatments and the wonderful care he received during his experience.

In his blog he says: "Also, very importantly, I've read blogs that related to my issues and I found them useful for what I was about to go through – if this helps one person through the process and makes others aware, then the effort to write it all down will be worth it."

Dan was prepared to share everything. His main mantras throughout were always positive: "It will all be fine," "Everything will be o.k." and "No matter the odds, never give up." The third one was said to him by a colleague, Craig, who lost his battle, but his words went on to become a part of Dan's family's mantra.

Dan's team mates all vouched for him, claiming that Nat had no future recourse on the rugby front from now on, as it was indeed thanks to the great game of rugby that Dan's life had been saved.

Might Make You Smile
NERF ATTACK

Susan was a thirty-something-year-old mum of two lively boys. Having been diagnosed with Breast Cancer, she had undergone all the treatments and was looking forward to getting her life back on track. With her family by her side, and her faith she knew she could withstand anything. Her cancer had taught her so many lessons. She felt she had found her 'real' friends, and was surprised that sometimes those she had thought were closest, had not always proven to be so. But Susan had also learnt that there was no right or wrong way to deal with the 'C' word and that everyone was entitled to their own approach.

She felt that she had gone through hell and back, as had her family, but now she wanted to focus on being 'normal' again. Her appearance wasn't by any means all-consuming, but she was the first to admit that her goal of feeling as much like her old self as possible did, to a degree, include how she looked.

There came the day when she was having the final touches to her breast reconstruction, and it was the time she had been truly looking forward to, she liked to call it "nipple time". Having had the breast reconstruction done in stages, this was literally the 'cherry on the cake'. Nipples were to be created and added to her already reconstructed, and much loved 'boobs'.

The morning came and the operation went off without a hitch. The specialist surgeon created the nipples and had attached them with infinite care and precision. Bound and dressed, Susan was glad to be going home to heal. This, to her, was the final stages of completing and surviving her cancer; and ultimately thriving as a woman, wife, and mother. She couldn't wait to see the end results. The surgeon had warned her that the dressings would be there for a time, it was vital she took things very slowly, and she adheres to her surgeon's words on how to help aid in her recovery. Susan couldn't wait for the day she could remove the dressings, she knew she would enjoy the great unveiling.

Life carried on with a home and family to look after. Susan was careful to keep her exertion to a minimum, and the whole family made fun of her for resembling a mummy with her dressings.

Susan waited patiently for the day when she could remove the final dressing. Being the mother of lively boys, she had learnt to dodge most missiles, glide over Lego, always be up for sporting licky, sticky tattoos to be stuck in various inappropriate places, and deal with pretty much everything her offspring had launched her way.

Getting dressed one morning she was a little slower than normal, and was momentarily taken by surprise by her youngest, liveliest son, who was currently in the guise of an elite assassin. Armed with a Nerf gun fully loaded with its foam-tipped bullets and safety catch off, she heard the sharp click and felt the ping before she could remove herself from its line of fire. Zap! The bullet had hit its intended target spot on. Mum had been got. The tiny assassin fled the scene of the crime with a drop and roll maneuver that James Bond would have been proud of, his mission had been accomplished.

What had actually been shot at, with perfect aim and precision, was one of her brand new, still settling themselves in, and already much loved nipples. As Susan looked downwards she already knew all was not well. She called for her husband – who as luck would have it was a paramedic – not long recovered from a long night shift, but fortunately home that day. He quickly came to the bedroom to find his wife attempting to reposition the much longed for nipple.

Her husband, being the more medically minded of the couple, knew what he had to do. Susan insisted she didn't want to go back to the specialist, stating that after such a long time with treatment upon treatment you only went to the hospital when you absolutely had to.

Between Susan and her husband, they lovingly and ever so carefully repositioned the nipple and he steri-stripped that little bud right back into place as best he could. Disaster, they hoped, had been diverted.

A while later, back at the hospital for the follow-up appointment with the surgeon who had performed Susan's procedure, Susan removed her top. She stood absolutely still, staring frontwards, hardly able to breathe. There followed a great deal of frowning and quizzical examinations of her breasts. Susan and her husband avoided eye contact with each other and the consultant. Susan held her breath for what seemed like an age. The surgeon finally gave his verdict; he wasn't happy with the alignment of the nipples and felt at least one should be redone. He did question how one nipple seemed somewhat misplaced and couldn't quite understand how it had come about.

Susan countered that she was in fact delighted with the results, and there was really no need to spend any more time on her breasts. After all, she was happy, healthy, and getting on with life; that was what mattered. Susan also pointed out that nobody had perfect breasts anyway; a little uniqueness added to the authenticity, and she shared a knowing smile with her husband. They then left the hospital for the last time.

Good For A Grin
MAN'S NATURAL POSE

Yes, Gareth was relaxed, slouched back on the sofa, hand down his pants cupping his nuts, watching T.V. in man's most natural pose. Mmm… something wasn't quite right down there. One was definitely larger than the other and not in the usual way, there was distinctive swelling. Something was up.

The next day Gareth sensibly took himself of to the docs. His wife's pleading was ringing in his ear: "Can you just tell them you found a lump, rather than sounding like some weird pervert?" Gareth, however, was all for authenticity: if he was lounging with his hand down his pants when making his discovery, so be it. Tell it as it is.

The doctor diagnosed an infection and made a non-urgent referral for four to six weeks. Unsatisfied, but in the usual, true, polite British manner, Gareth said "Thank you very much" and left.

As is often the case at these sort of times, Gareth quickly came to his senses and marched straight back into the surgery. A little shouting, and possibly accompanied by some gesticulating (we all know the details become vague when the red mist falls) later he was granted an urgent referral. Probably given partly in the hope of getting him to leave the premises quicker, but he had the urgent referral nonetheless.

His diagnosis for testicular cancer was confirmed and bollock removal (orchidectomy) surgery was scheduled.

By the time the day for the surgery arrived, Gareth and his wife had welcomed their new baby, Finley, and been immersed in the craziness and the full sleep-deprived existence of parenting for two weeks – they were exhausted. At the hospital, Gareth was on his bed in the pre-operative waiting area – his wife saw her opportunity for much needed sleep, (new baby remember) and climbed onto the bed and under the covers. In no time the couple drifted off into a deep sleep.

They were woken by the surgeon, who frankly couldn't get over how "relaxed" Gareth was about the procedure. Parent of a beautiful baby boy, wife snuggled up beside him – losing a nut was hardly going to put too much of a dampener on things.

Might Make You Smile
BALL BEARING BRACELET

Kay loved her bracelets. There were three of them made of silver, and they held charms that she had collected which signified the momentous events of her life: from having children, wedding anniversaries, and everything in-between. She wore the bracelets often and loved all that they represented.

Kay was well-known as the sort of person who could make a dull day bright. She had an uncanny knack for cheering up those around her, and possessed a wicked sense of fun and humour. It was Kay people went to when they were down; her positivity shone through, and you couldn't help but smile when you met her. She worked in an old-people's home and loved her job. The residents adored her creativity, and nothing was ever too much trouble for her.

As she was undergoing tests and scans for her diagnosed breast cancer, she had to have ball bearings placed on her breasts for one particular procedure, a guided wire mammogram. She smiled to herself as she had an idea. The procedures seemed to take forever, but when they were finally over she pulled the consultant to one side. At first he thought he had misheard and asked Kay to repeat herself. She slowly and deliberately stated her request once more. The consultant was a little taken aback, but then smiled and said he would have to speak to various people; he would get back to her.

During her next appointment, Kay left the consultant's office smiling to herself. The ball bearings that had been used in the scan, now have pride of place on bracelet number three.

Kay loves to show off her bracelet and watch people's reactions when she explains the significance of the ball bearings. She has survived breast cancer, and she loves to look at the ball bearings as a reminder of what she has gone through and how she loves her life. They now share a place alongside all the other great and important events of her life. Kay also loves the shock value of them; they never fail to make people smile.

Good For A Grin
LIFE IS A ROLLERCOASTER

Mike had his suspicions. Trips to the bathroom throughout the night, nothing new there, but when instead of pee he noticed there was blood, the voice inside his head told him it was time to get things checked out.

He did just that. Unfortunately the timing of the discovery was not the greatest. Mike and his wife Ann were in the process of challenging a district council 120 miles away from where they lived concerning council tax on their apartment on the coast. They had an appointment to meet a council representative and really didn't want to miss it, but the health issue was acute.

The decision between Mike and his wife was to make an appointment with their G.P. and take it from there. At the appointment that morning, the G.P. asked Mike what he thought the problem was. He explained his thoughts were that it was either something or nothing. Mike had, however, been concerned with the threat of cancer – it had been at the back of his mind for the past ten years or so, having had so many relatives die from the disease. The G.P. was very understanding, neither alarmist nor understating the possible situation.

Various blood tests were booked. The conveyor belt had started. After the tests, there were appointments at Addenbrooke's within the following two weeks. Mike's anxieties rose during this time. The obvious questions, 'Have I got cancer?', 'Yes' and 'No' were bouncing around his head, the stakes rising higher and higher.

Kidneys and bladder were scanned, cystoscopy performed, and, lastly prostate palpitated. Mike felt something during the palpitation. The consultant explained things looked clear but that there was a nodule; it could just have been harmless but he would take the results to the Multi-Disciplinary Team and get back to him with the outcome.

Mike and his wife shared their concerns. Ann's first husband had died of cancer at seventy, so here she was again with a similar possibility. She and Mike were able to support each other as the conveyor belt of tests, scans and appointments continued. Life, as is always the case, still carried on. Dealing with other issues was both a distraction and sometimes an inconvenience.

Trying to focus and concentrate on daily activities was difficult. Ann and Mike decided they would tell their families as an M.R.I. scan appointment was getting closer and they would need help from their children taking care of things, including Ann's mum, who was in a care home.

Mike received a 'Summary of Pending Results and Final Plan, in the post. He read cytology benign (normal) and was ecstatic, he was free from cancer. He quickly sent an email to all friends and family and even his G.P. to that effect. He was on a high, life could get back to being normal. He had had a scare but all was well.

Two days later Mike got a telephone call. It was the cancer nurse specialist (obviously to confirm the good news). What he actually heard was that he had a grade five growth. A grade five growth was highly suspicious. Mike explained he had received the report stating 'cytology benign (normal)'. "Ahh, you're reading the urine sample results," she said. The nurse went on to explain there was in fact the possibility he did have cancer.

The anxieties rose to new heights. The conveyor belt was about to pick up pace again. He felt so alone, cold, and remembered an advert he had seen on the television for Macmillan nurses – the man was alone in a hospital gown in a barren landscape. He could completely relate to it.

Bizarrely, it was at that point that his humour came to the fore. He caught himself saying to nobody in particular: "There's no need to go to Alton Towers, I'm getting a rollercoaster ride for nothing, it's all on the NHS!" Up and down, round and round, up and down again, the emotions never seemed to stop. He had to smile to himself, his sense of humour was still intact, if slightly warped. Hardly surprising, but still there nonetheless.

Might Make You Smile
HAIR TODAY, GONE TONIGHT

June may have been in her seventies, but she still loved to go out, socialise, and enjoy herself. Her cancer treatments often meant that she wasn't always able to do the things she loved to do; she was not always feeling well enough. When the good days came, and June could go out with her friends and partner, she loved nothing more than going out for a drink or to dinner for the evening.

It was a "good" day, and June was looking forward to going out that night with her partner. The cancer treatments had meant that June had lost her hair, but she had decided she would wear a wig that night. She didn't often wear one, feeling more comfortable without, but she felt she would make the effort that evening. She was pleased with the result in the mirror and was looking forward to an evening of fun. Her new glossy hair swished around her shoulders, and the fringe gave her a whole new glamorous look. June was feeling like a million dollars.

June, her partner, and friends had chosen a lively pub for the evening. She was soaking up the atmosphere; everyone seemed to be on good form, and she was enjoying herself. After a couple of drinks, a friend leant towards June, being deaf, June read her lips. She could see that her friend was suggesting she go to the ladies. Somewhat puzzled, June followed her friend to the toilets.

Pushing open the heavy door, June gasped as she saw her reflection in the mirror. The wig had slid completely to one side, and the fringe was by her chin. One minute June was laughing at the ridiculousness of her reflection, the next she was cross that none of her party had mentioned anything sooner. The more she looked at her reflection the more she laughed, she decided she looked more like an obscure version of 'Cousin Itt' from the Addams Family than anything else. She straightened her wig and returned to the bar, but it was at that point June decided wigs were not for her. Although she kept the wig on until the end of the evening she acknowledged she felt much more 'herself' once the hairpiece was tucked away in her bag at the end of the night.

As much as June enjoyed the glamour of the wig, she wasn't sure if she enjoyed the laughter her 'Cousin Itt' impersonation brought her and her friends more.

June has never worn a wig again and she still berates her friends for not informing her sooner of her 'wardrobe malfunction'. Even now, she cannot finish telling the story without bursting out laughing thinking of the absurdity of her reflection in the mirror that night. Proving wigs are not for all, and certainly not for June.

Good For A Grin
FOR THE LOVE OF RUGBY

Ben could hear the pounding of booted feet behind him. He was so close to the touchline he could almost taste it.

His heart was racing, the try was his. He just had to reach out as his arm extended and put the ball firmly in place. Control of the movement was all-important, all he could think of was "Don't drop the ball, don't drop the ball."

The pain was the first thing he registered, a searing, burning, take your breath away pain that was so severe it rendered him speechless. Perhaps a better description would be soundless. He wanted to scream, yell, whatever, but the shock of the severity of the pain seemed to have rendered him incapable.

"Sorry mate, you ok?" The opposition team member was looking down at Ben. Ben was still incapable of moving. His hands had naturally gone to his testicles, where the damage had been done. He waited for the pain to subside and catch his breath.

Eventually he was able to get up, though the pain was still an eleven on the one-to-ten scale. The try had been awarded. Ben was delighted, if not incredibly sore. Limping off the pitch, he couldn't believe the pain was still so strong. The beers that followed the game helped a little, however.

The following morning, Ben was still very sore and hugely swollen. He told himself it was all due to the smack 'down there' he had been on the receiving end of during the match. But he was aware the swelling didn't look like it was going down. Thinking it best to get it checked out, he went to hospital, still putting everything down to the rugby accident. Scans were ordered and completed.

There was a little niggle at the back of his mind that was kept there by the old "It will never happen to me" adage.

After numerous scans and appointments Ben got the news he had dreaded, he had testicular cancer. The issue was with Ben's right testicle and it needed to be removed. The date for the operation was made.

Ben arrived at the hospital and waited to meet the surgeon. She came into the consulting room. "So, let's have a look at this LEFT testicle that's been giving you all these problems," she said as she knelt down in front of Ben. "Actually, the problem is with the right testicle," Ben replied. He quickly dropped his shorts. The surgeon took his testicles in her hands for examination. "Oh, yes!" she said. "You are quite right. That's lucky, we could have taken the wrong one!"

Ben wasn't quite sure how he felt about her remark. He was, however, very relieved when he came round from the operation, lifted the bed sheet and discovered the right one had gone and the left one was left.

Might Make You Smile
A NIGHT OUT WITH KYLIE

Kylie was the name given to Clare's newly acquired, highly fashionable, and fabulously glossy wig. Even though Clare came from a family of fashion and beauty conscious hairdressing females, she had adapted to her hair loss during her cancer treatment pretty quickly. She had, in fact, found it character building. In the grand scheme of things a little hair loss was not something she concerned herself with.

However, Clare did, on occasion, take Kylie out. With a night out coming up, Clare decided she would wear Kylie. With a final check of her appearance and with Kylie firmly in place, Clare was ready for some fun.

A great night of chatting, eating, drinking, and plenty of laughter was exactly what Clare enjoyed. Soon it was time to leave, and everyone was saying their goodbyes. Clare went round the group hugging everyone, In mid-hug with one particular friend Clare felt an odd sensation; Kylie was on the move! Unfortunately, the beautiful bracelet worn by her friend had become caught in Kylie, and the much-admired wig was slowly making its way off Clare's head and heading toward her shoulders. The bracelet wearing friend was mortified; the restaurant was full and the incident was sure to have been noticed by the other diners. Clare couldn't help but laugh as Kylie and the bracelet were separated. It took all of her reassurances, between fits of giggles, to mollify her friend, then her friend finally began to see the funny side. Clare joked that Kylie had always had the capability to draw plenty of attention.

Good For A Grin
PREGGERS?...

On October 24th, James was diagnosed with testicular cancer. He had noticed a lump and had taken himself off to the doctors, to be told it was nothing to worry about.

Two more weeks passed and James realised the lump wasn't getting any smaller. He was pondering his predicament when he recalled reading a story a few years previously about a guy who had, as a joke, taken a pregnancy test and it showed up positive. Being somewhat gobsmacked, the man had looked into the result further, it being not exactly expected, and it transpired he had cancer! James decided he would do the same thing. He got exactly the same result. James ,according to the 'stick', was pregnant!

The next day James went to the doctor, who got him to take another test. The same thing happened. James was definitely pregnant! The reason for this phenomenon is that when women are pregnant they produce a hormone that can also be found in some testicular cancers.

Within a day, James was at the hospital to have the findings confirmed. He did in fact have cancer.

The following week, James was admitted to have the operation to remove his right testicle (orchidectomy). A painful couple of weeks recovering followed. The operation was a success, and after a time James was able to return to work.

As is often the case there will be future scans and appointments, all helping to keep an eye on things. From the strangest of findings James was diagnosed and treated. He was very impressed with the level of care he received and deeply grateful to all the doctors and nurses involved. It is their care we rely on, after all.

So, fellas, should you be inclined and choose to pee on that stick, rest assured you won't be the first.

Might Make You Smile
MR & MRS SALT AND PEPPER POT

When Mrs Salt was diagnosed with cancer and lost her hair very quickly due to her chemotherapy, it was initially distressing for her, but she came to terms with it and life carried on, as it so often does. It was only when Mr and Mrs Salt's children were getting confused by their parents' appearance from the back, that the Salt's came up with an ingenious plan. Mrs Salt didn't like the feel of a hairpiece or wig, they made her hot and uncomfortable, she was never able to keep it on straight, and it felt like she was wearing a hat all the time – which wasn't particularly her style either. As busy as she was at home, she felt they just seemed to get in her way, so she decided to wear nothing.

Mr Salt had been bald all his adult life and that was no big deal until Mrs Salt's diagnosis and subsequent treatment. From the back, the little Salt's were becoming confused, they couldn't always tell their parents apart; often thinking they were calling out to dad when in fact they were talking to mum and vice-versa. The frustrations of the Salt family were heightened when the children would demand school uniforms and packed lunches from a fearful looking Mr Salt; who didn't know where to start looking for such mysterious items. would panic, and run to find Mrs Salt.

Mr and Mrs Salt were at home together one day while the little Salts were at school, and they came up with a marvellous plan. Mrs Salt found a thick eyeshadow pencil in a chocolate brown shade. Mr Salt wrote on the back of Mrs Salt's head 'MUM' in neat, large letters. In turn, Mrs Salt wrote on the back of Mr Salt's head 'DAD'. The little Salts came home from school that day and were delighted with their parent's efforts; harmony was restored in the Salt household.

The Salts were able to adapt their heads for an upcoming Fancy Dress Party by simply adding one single circle in the centre of Mrs Salt's head, and three circles on Mr Salt's head. Mr and Mrs Salt went to the Fancy Dress as salt and pepper pots. Not only did they delight their children with their creativity, they won first prize at the Fancy Dress Party.

Good For A Grin
OH WHAT A NIGHT!

Nick's discovery of his testicular cancer came about in a somewhat unorthodox way. A thirty-one-year-old single dad, working as a police officer, juggling life and after a very successful night out with a lovely lady (no beer goggle disaster there) discovers he is a little 'tender' the following morning. Upon closer inspection he noticed a small lump on his left testicle and it was a little painful to touch.

While getting the results from having a growth removed from his neck, Nick had mentioned the lump on his testicle, pants down. A few more questions were asked about Nick's medical history, and when he mentioned he had had an operation to descend a testicle when he was ten, the doctor straight away sent him for an ultrasound scan. Pants up.

Pants down again, Nick asked the radiographer if she could tell him what was going on. He explained he didn't mean to be awkward or was going to get angry, he just would really like to know what was happening.. She was a lovely lady and showed him the scan. It was obvious there was something on the left testicle that didn't look right. Pants up and back to the doctor again. Dropping his pants once more, Nick realised it was becoming second nature by now; interesting habit to have, he mused.

At the doctors, he was told he would receive the full results the following week. It was a few days later that Nick was asked to St. James Hospital, Leeds. At the hospital, the discussion of further children in the future came up and it was recommended that a sperm sample be deposited. Nick considered this a fair point.

Finding the department where this was to be done, he walked into a very large and busy main waiting area.

There were a number of other people there for various other appointments. It was obvious they were certainly not all there for the same reason as Nick. His name was called, and he was somewhat ceremoniously handed a cup and shown to a room. Pants down again. When the deposit had been made, was Nick able to leave discreetly by a separate exit with his dignity intact? Did a nurse quietly knock on the door and remove the sample for him? Unfortunately not – Nick had to take his sample, cup in hand, straight back to the main reception and hand it over in front of a waiting room full of people. Yes, it was obvious to all exactly what he had been up to.

There was no other cause of action to take, other than to smile sweetly and walk with definite purpose out of the waiting room.

Might Make You Smile
NOT MY FINEST HOUR

Jo had always been someone who you could have written a thousand amusing stories about her. An intelligent woman who had a flare for art and design and loved dogs, cats, and every other animal you could imagine. Jo was a woman to whom a lot of things happened to. She had some amazing stories about events that were almost too incredible to believe, but you knew they were actually true. If there were ever to be a stampeding herd of wildebeest rampaging through the countryside, the spectacle would have happened in Jo's neck of the woods; and it would have been nothing unusual if they had targeted Jo's beautiful garden to charge through. There had been lost dogs, chickens, even donkeys, wandering the country lanes and it was to Jo's house they headed for. Her friends loved her dearly anyway, but all the more for her regaling of an average day in her life.

Jo was diagnosed with cancer in December, and after numerous consultations and surgeries, her radiotherapy treatment was to begin in March. Prior to the treatment there were various scans and tests to be carried out. Jo had been given an appointment for an early morning scan and had set her alarm clock accordingly to allow for plenty of time to get to the hospital.

The day did not start well. The alarm did not go off and Jo, who had been unable to sleep properly for weeks (another symptom of her cancer), had slept soundly all night. When she finally woke, she knew instinctively she was late. As luck would have it, she also acknowledged she was having a 'bad' day because her energy levels were already low. Added to this, was her ability to only locate antique knickers of an undecipherable shade and no bra – it had inexplicably disappeared in the space of twelve hours. She suspected one of the family dogs but had no time or energy to track down the culprit. She quickly resigned herself to having to go out with only fifty percent of her underwear, reasoning she would have probably had to remove the item anyway for the scan. On time, notwithstanding a household search, she left for the hospital only to hit rush hour traffic almost immediately.

Sitting in traffic, Jo seized the opportunity. She delved quickly into her bag in an attempt to at least locate a hairbrush to try and tame her wayward head of thick, curly hair which had amassed itself into an impressive "bedhead" beehive hairdo. It was then that she realised she had in fact picked up the wrong bag and was minus any cosmetics or grooming paraphernalia. Jo scooped out the crumby contents of the bag onto the passenger seat, only to find a couple of hairy, slightly gooey Haribo sweets, and a long forgotten, possibly unpaid, parking ticket.

Eventually arriving at the hospital, she was shown into her cubicle and given a gown to wear during her scan. Cursing the bralessness of her upper body, the skimpiness of the gown, and its inability to barely meet where it should, but congratulating herself on guessing correctly that she would be asked to remove the garment anyway. She cursed to herself once more about the shapelessness and dubious shade of her knickers, only adding to her less than glamorous appearance when she bolted upright, startled by a knock on her cubicle door. The surprise of the knock found her banging her head with some force on the shoe shelf above, and then stubbing her toe while in the process of trying to open the cubicle door. Unable to stop the torrent of colourful expletives blurting from her mouth, in walks "Dr Drop-Dead Gorgeous." A man at least ten years her junior, broad-shouldered, and looking like he stepped off the set of E.R. or Grey's Anatomy. As well as greeting her doctor red-faced, foul-mouthed, bare-chested, and rubbing her head, Jo also happened to notice that the large clock on the wall behind him was showing it was ten-thirty. The day had hardly begun.

Good For A Grin
MIKE'S MAD DASH

Mike had discovered a lump on his testicle. He knew he had to be proactive and get it checked out as soon as possible. He was a father of one and expecting his second child any day now. His family was everything to him. It would have been the easiest thing to wait until the new arrival was there and then get things looked into, but he was also aware that these things needed to be acted on quickly – time was of the essence.

Admittedly, with his wife heavily pregnant the timing could have been better, but that is just the way life is. Within two weeks his operation was scheduled, Mike had testicular cancer and his testicle needed to be removed.

Life threw him another curve ball as he was having his operation at Pinderfields Hospital – his wife went into labour at Dewsbury and District Hospital in Wakefield.

As soon as Mike came round from his operation he was off making his uncomfortable way to Dewsbury to be with his wife. He arrived to see his daughter being born, and thanks to his quick actions and resulting early detection, he is now enjoying watching his two daughters grow up.

Mike is a member of Battling Fat Lads football team. They are sponsored by the OddBalls Foundation and raise money through charity football matches. They are also regular competitors in the FA People's Cup.

Might Make You Smile
PAMMIES

Being in her sixties, Ina found that fashion had skipped past her. She was happy to pick up on perhaps the odd one or two styles, but no longer had the desperate need to be completely up to date with her wardrobe. She was now happy to be comfortable above all else.

She liked to think she watched her weight and was careful in the amount of wine she consumed; she liked to think that, but reality didn't always match up. Nevertheless, she was a lady who knew life was for living, and that a little overindulgence every now and then was good for the soul.

The tiniest pinprick of blood on the inside of her bra cup was the only indication Ina had that there was the very faint possibility that something wasn't quite right. Thanks to quick action on her and her doctor's part, produced the positive test results revealed during a follow-up appointment that Ina had breast cancer. Although shocked and a little scared, Ina was a woman of common sense and cast iron will; she was prepared for the treatments that would come next.

After a double mastectomy and chemotherapy, she already considered herself to be on the home stretch of her 'run-in' with cancer, which was how she preferred to think of her illness; a blip that life throws you from time-to-time. It was only when the reconstruction surgery was discussed and finally scheduled that she gave any thought to her appearance. Ina was surprised at how her opinion of herself had subtly changed.

Suddenly she was shopping for summer clothes; off the shoulder dresses and strappy sun tops. Ina had a vision of something in her mind that she had never considered before. She knew there was one thing she now craved more than anything, a red one-piece swimming costume. Ina kept her longing a secret. She planned a grand unveiling, poolside, on the next family holiday.

Finding a one-piece in bright red took almost as long as the completion of the reconstruction surgery itself. On a cold March morning while browsing in a department store, she came across the longed for item. Finding a size to fit had been a minor issue. The assistant rang the supplier who confirmed that although there was not a demand for that particular size, they did stock them, and one would be sent over with the next delivery.

Ina recovered from all the surgery and treatments; she had lost a little weight but not so much to make a difference in her wardrobe. The day Ina's consultant gave her the great news that she was well again, was only a couple of months before the family holiday. Ina's excitement grew with every passing day running up to her longed for holiday.

The sun beat down intensely as Ina and three generations of her family touched down in Spain. The villa was perfect, with a huge pool, enormous gardens and terraces, and enough room for all of the grandchildren to run around and have a great time. With bags unpacked and swimming costumes on, everyone made their way down to the pool. Ina kept her sarong tied in the style of a dress so as to not spoil her unveiling. When everyone was in the pool Ina untied her sarong. The grandchildren cheered and clapped, Ina's children who were grown up and with children of their own, bobbed around open mouthed staring at their mother in shock, and then they too whooped and clapped.

"If Nannie's got to have pammies, then she'll have the swimming costume to match." Ina laughed as she struck a slow-motion running pose, just like Pamela Anderson in Baywatch. The red swimming costume, and Ina's new figure, was laughed and talked about all holiday by the whole family. From that moment on Ina's breasts were known to all as her 'pammies', and the red swimming costume became a family legend.

Good For A Grin
BOWEL MOVEMENTS AND PEEING

So, as with so many medical events, when diagnosing and being diagnosed with cancer, whatever type of cancer it is, the age-old questions come into play.

"Do you poo regularly?", "How often do you poo?", "Have you noticed any changes in your poo?"

Same goes for peeing. "Do you find you have the urge to pee more?", "What colour is your pee?", "How much, roughly, do you think you pee?"

Now, from a male point of view, peeing, farting and pooing are all perfect fodder for comedy and regaling, bringing forth a great deal of merriment; but when it comes down to taking much more serious notice of these things, no, it is not always top of our agenda.

Did we have a skinfull Saturday night after the England rugby match? Yes, yes we did. Did I pee a lot? Of course. Was it closely followed by a much anticipated chicken vindaloo, Bombay potatoes and hot pickle-eating contest? Yes, yes it was. Did I poo a lot? You betcha!

You can see how hard it can be for the average male to even contemplate a change in either of these habits. We barely take notice of them normally.

It usually takes something dramatic to make us notice something. Only when this 'notice' has been taken do things move forward.

So my advice would be; after reading this, for a couple of days just take a little more notice of what your body does.

Yes, stare at that poo (no, it is not necessary to poke it with a stick, leave that to the medical profession, should they choose), notice how often you pee. Pay a bit more attention to your body. It might just help you notice something you may have missed.

Might Make You Smile
WHITE VAN MAN

Sadie had tried to keep her hair as straight and neat as possible, but the warm summer weather was making it difficult. Keeping the beautifully cut and styled ash blonde wig straight and in place was not easy.

It was a hot summer's day, and although the studio was air-conditioned, the amount of equipment used to keep the radio station going meant there was still heat emitting around her desk. The drugs she was taking as part of her cancer treatment also meant her internal 'temperature gauge', as she liked to call it, was often on the blink. Sometimes she fluctuated from being excessively hot and then very cold, usually at inappropriate times.

On this particular day, she could already feel her head was molten beneath the mesh of the hairpiece. Her fingers felt under the hair and touched the soft fuzziness of her own regrowth. Sadie knew it would be a few more months before her own hair would be noticeable again, and she often wondered what colour it would come back as. With the heat beneath the wig intensifying and making her uncomfortable, Sadie counted down the ten minutes left of the radio show and longed for the time when she could make her way home and walk in the fresh air.

She finished up with a good laugh with a listener who had called in to tell the story of how his cat had run around with a small bird in its mouth for half an hour while being madly chased by the owner. Upon capture, the owner found that what he thought to be a fowl was, in fact, the remnants of his dinner of sausages, pinched from his plate while he had gone to answer the telephone.

Leaving the radio station, Sadie stepped out into the sunshine. The crossing outside the studio was busy; lunchtime meant an increase in the traffic, and there was a crossroad junction immediately off a large roundabout. Sadie's head was really beginning to itch and feel doubly uncomfortable, stepping out onto the crossing she couldn't bear it any longer. In a single movement, she grabbed the wig and plucked it from her head. Then followed a series of unexpected events.

The sound of car horns used in anger and the screeching of brakes filled the air. Sadie turned, enjoying the deliciousness of the cool air against her scalp and was smiling as she turned. It was then that she saw the large white van, which had stopped abruptly at the crossing. Its passengers, she guessed, were builders judging by the writing emblazoned on all the surfaces of the van. She registered three expressions of absolute shock; mouths wide open, eyes bulging, and looking directly at her. She could also hear a strange sound, it was the yell of disbelief emanating from each of the open mouths, "Whoa Mrs!". It took a moment for Sadie to realise that the rest of the traffic commotion was due to the van straddling two lanes. Its occupants had obviously stopped the van sharply having seen a blonde haired lady effectively scalp herself in broad daylight.

Sadie was unable to help herself; she was laughing as she apologised profusely to the van's clearly traumatised occupants and the other traffic that had been forced to stop suddenly. She explained she was absolutely fine and that there was nothing to worry about; trying desperately not to laugh at the burly men who were still clearly shocked by what they had seen. Enjoying the coolness of the summer air, Sadie made her way home laughing loudly to herself every time she pictured the three faces in the white van.

Good For A Grin
P.E.T. SCAN MEETS RADIOACTIVE MAN

Blue? Seriously, blue pee? When you have already been told you need to stay clear of pregnant women and children (Not 'pregnant children', in case you were wondering) after having a P.E.T. scan. Blue pee, to boot, had to be seen to be believed. Dave had to smile though as he watched the blue liquid circle the toilet bowl.

Did he feel like a five-year-old boy again, able to glean some amusement and fascination from unusual toilet habits? Yes, yes he did. Did he wish he could share the moment with half a dozen of his mates, who he knew would be equally fascinated and fully appreciate the spectacle? Yes, yes he did.

The knock at the door and the nurse's voice asking if he was okay brought him back from his reverie. "Are you okay in there Dave?"

"Fine, thanks nurse." He didn't think the nurse would be as fascinated as he was with his colourful accomplishments. . Having been told to flush twice, to make sure all radioactive residue was dispelled, Dave made his way back to the cubicle.

He had been given a list of precautionary things he needed to know about after his scan. Dave felt a little bit like a pioneer, having to break new ground in science with his radioactivity and azure emissions. In truth, he knew many had gone before him, doing exactly the same thing, but he enjoyed the moment for what it was. Peeing on command (as was required after the actual scan) had never been an issue for Dave and he was somewhat pleased with himself that he could empty his bladder as and when commanded. This was accompanied by much praise from the radiographer.

The precautions varied from keeping bodily fluids away from others, changing bed sheets if necessary and the need for glove-wearing nursing staff. Dave allowed his imagination to take over, visions of himself in steel worker mode, wearing elbow-length industrial gloves, a rubber smock apron, and full-face welding mask, popped into his head, looking somewhat similar to the executioner from one of the Black Adder series. In reality, light disposable gloves were worn by the nurses with nothing for him (he was, after all, the 'radioactive' one).

Having read something somewhere that a P.E.T. scan might set off radiation alarms at airports, Dave discovered he had almost an all-consuming urge to test this theory at the nearest one. Fortunately, the nearest was hours away.

Dave, when he was back in the comfort of his chair, beside his bed, scan completed and enjoying a cup of tea, came to the conclusion that being diagnosed with cancer had, among other things, made him more creative in his thinking and had reignited a somewhat neglected mischievous side to his nature. He felt this needed to be both embraced and exploited. Yes, it could be time to have a little fun, he mused. Look out, world.

Might Make You Smile
GREEN WITH ENVY, NOT SO MUCH...

Michelle was late for work. It didn't seem to matter how much earlier she set the alarm, time appeared to elude her. She could have blamed it on the effects of the chemotherapy treatment for her ovarian cancer, but she never did. Sometimes she just didn't feel like herself, but she managed to shake that feeling by the time she got to the office.

Working was not for everyone who was experiencing life with cancer, but for Michelle it was important on many levels. It was something she had always done – been a hard worker – so when she became ill she tried her best to fit in work around it and the subsequent treatments. Unfortunately, the cancer returned on an almost annual basis and each time Michelle dealt with it with a re-newed stoicism. She often liked to joke that her husband had a new woman every year for probably the last five years. The chemotherapy treatment had meant the loss of her hair, but each time it had grown back it had come through a different colour and texture, it had been straight, curly, thick, and thin.

Michelle had found wearing a wig something that had become a bit of a routine; as had remembering to pencil on eyebrows every morning. She often felt it was the eyebrows more than anything that completed and framed a face, giving it definition. Afterall, with so many different hairstyles and accessories that could cover a head, hair sometimes went almost unseen. Hats, scarves, and headbands all aided in covering or filling in what was actually on top of your head, but eyebrows are just there on the front of the face and taken for granted, but definitely missed when they are gone.

Michelle looked at the clock once more, again it had lurched forward dramatically, and she was definitely on the late side now. Quickly, she pencilled on the well-practiced arch over each eye. Grabbing her shoes, and her favourite bag, she made a dash for the front door.

The railway station was abuzz with the low rumble of commuters; who were waiting to be crammed like sardines on the train to Liverpool Street Station. There were many familiar faces, and all were smiling in Michelle's direction as she boarded the train. She was fortunate enough to get a seat sitting opposite a middle aged man reading the daily newspaper. He acknowledged her with a nod and, with what Michelle thought was a quizzical look. She wondered if he thought he recognised her from somewhere, but he certainly didn't seem familiar to her.

The train finally pulled into Liverpool Street Station. Michelle could feel her mouth becoming dry, as often happened; another side effect of the drugs used in her treatment. She needed to buy some water and a packet of chewing gum, she knew this would help alleviate the problem, so she headed for the nearest newsagent. Standing in line waiting to pay, Michelle was becoming increasingly aware of people's stares. Strangers were looking in her direction, their gazes lingering just a fraction too long. She was beginning to feel a little self-conscious and checked her outfit. She was wearing a smart business suit, check; no holes in tights, check; matching shoes, check; nothing seemed out of place.

As soon as she reached her office building, she headed straight to the ladies toilets. Under the harsh, bright lights, it became gloriously obvious to her why her appearance had caused so much interest. As expertly as her eyebrows were drawn on, there was one small detail she hadn't noticed while hurriedly doing her make-up that morning. The pencil she had used was not her usual soft brown shade. No, today she was sporting what could only be described as an almost metallic emerald shade, with plenty of sparkle. It was fair to say she would not have looked out of place as an extra on any science-fiction blockbuster film set. Laughing at her reflection, she promised herself she would pay more attention when applying her make-up, especially in the gloom of early mornings.

Good For A Grin
PUMP NO.1 AND PUMP NO.2

Fred was having a hard time dealing with the after-effects of his prostatectomy. For many men the two main problems are incontinence and E.D., the abbreviation for erectile dysfunction.

Fred had been made very aware of these issues prior to his surgery, but reading information leaflets, articles online and anything he could get his hands on was all very well – living with these issues day-to-day was a whole different matter. Fred was a man who possessed a great sense of humour and was always one to give advice along the lines of 'get it done, get it sorted, move on with life', always accompanied with a huge smile and a slap on the back. He found he was now having difficulty taking his own advice.

The euphoria – yes, that's right, euphoria – of having his surgery and knowing the biggest part of his encounter with prostate cancer had now been removed (a large tumour attached to the prostate), had now worn off. He had also been warned again that this was often the case. Alas, a warning is just that, a warning. Fred realised fairly quickly he needed help. He knew if he could get assistance with the physical side of his rehabilitation, then his emotional and mental wellbeing would follow suit. Coming to terms with this realisation made him ponder if this was in fact the 'male way' of dealing with things. If he were able to cope and ultimately flourish with the physical side of life, he felt maybe a man's mental wellbeing could be all the easier to bring into line.

The incontinence was a particular issue and Fred wanted it sorted. At meetings with his consultant and medical team, an artificial sphincter was discussed, the procedure involving a sphincter being placed around the urethra, with the central pump placed in the scrotum. To aid with erectile disfunction, and at around the same time, it was suggested that a cylinder be placed in the penis, a reservoir inserted into the abdomen and a pump placed in the scrotum.

Fred thought about all this information very carefully. In the midst of this he burst out laughing, perhaps not the best time, being in the consulting room, but he had to explain. It really wouldn't do to get the two pumps mixed up.

Ultimately, Fred chose neither option. A regiment of patience and his own brand of 'self-training', learning to predict his body's needs, establishing good routines and perseverance, helped him in the end.

Might Make You Smile
TAKE AIM, FIRE!

Jan thought she had got away with most of the possible, even predictable, side effects that her cancer treatment could bestow. That was until she was hit by unrelenting nausea, the inability to keep anything down, even water, and the feeling of absolute exhaustion. She tried desperately to put on a brave face, but it was becoming increasingly obvious that she was on the verge of dehydration and that her strength had been severely affected by the inability to eat anything.

Jan resigned herself to the fact that she would need to be admitted to hospital. It was a tough decision to make but it was one Jan had always known could happen. She hated more than anything leaving her family, but it was their insistence that she get some medication, rest, and sustenance, that made her brave enough to make the call.

Jan put on a good show of being upbeat and positive about going into hospital, she didn't want to worry the loved ones around her, but she admitted to herself she was feeling terrible. Once tucked up in bed, in what was lovingly referred to as The Penthouse Suite – actually being the top floor of Addenbrook's Hospital – and settled in with I.V.s for hydration and drugs to help with her symptoms, she was finally able to get some rest. The nausea however was unrelenting, and she was truly grateful when sleep finally came.

Jan woke to the sound of some sort of alarm. Panicking, she checked her pumps and I.V. lines, but everything looked fine, and the noise didn't seem to be coming from any of her equipment.

It was at that exact moment that she realised the sound was the buzzer announcing visiting time, simultaneously she experienced a powerful wave of nausea that completely engulfed her. She was powerless, and as if in slow motion she projectile vomited. She watched in horror as the contents of her stomach arched midair, and landed almost perfectly into her open handbag situated at the end of her bed.

At that very same moment, Jan could hear with crystal clarity, "Nice shot mum!" It was the unmistakable voice of her son, the whole family had come to visit her. It was unanimously agreed that Jan could not have performed the feat again if she tried. Jan bade a fond farewell to her handbag, there was to be no resurrection for it from that onslaught. Ironically, that was the last time Jan was sick; it was agreed it was a grand finale for sure.

Good For A Grin
SUCK IT IN, TENSE IT UP, WINDMILL IT IN

Examinations for anything medical can and always will be daunting, even nerve-wracking. However, when it comes to your 'bits' it's a whole new level. Just when you want to at least give a good show of yourself, everything shrinks away and often refuses to co-operate.

On one particular occasion Gareth found himself wearing only his socks, a truly sexy look for anyone, it's got to be said, very The Graduate. Wanting to make the most of his 'assets', he was putting himself through some lunges and stretches in his allotted examination room. The stretches were then accompanied by some vigorous 'windmilling' to make his somewhat shrivelled penis look bigger before 'presenting' to the consultant. Yes, this morning he was really putting himself through his paces.

If preparing for an intimate examination of 'the old fella' was an Olympic sport, on this day Gareth could well have qualified for Team GB.

The gods, however, were not smiling down on him on this particular day. He found himself doing the very thing he had laughed at men doing on beaches when an attractive girl sauntered by. Guilty as charged, Gareth was putting in a mammoth effort, holding in his stomach and tensing every single muscle while the very attractive, Italian, female consultant carefully examined him. Let's just say 'awkward!'

Might Make You Smile
HELP, SHARK!

Vera was a proud grandmother, and loved to fill her time with doing as much as possible with her grandchildren. Even before she received the diagnosis of breast cancer, she would take them swimming at the local swimming pool every Sunday and then they would all return home to enjoy Sunday lunch together.

Vera had known in her heart that something wasn't quite right; she hadn't been feeling one hundred percent. Then she discovered a small lump, no bigger than a pea, in her left breast. A short time after, she had been diagnosed with breast cancer. The biggest blow to come to terms with initially was the lack of energy she had, and the fact that she missed out on the time spent with her grandchildren.

Vera's treatment went on longer than she had expected and her recovery hit a few bumps in the road, but slowly she began to feel stronger. The surgery to remove both breasts had been hard to come to terms with and she felt she wanted to pause before considering any further reconstructive surgery. She opted for prosthetic breast implants that were worn inside custom made underwear and even swimwear. Vera eventually got the hang of wearing her 'additions' and although not ideal, they did give her the confidence to do the everyday things she had always loved to do.

After a time, Vera felt confident enough to start taking her grandchildren swimming again at the local pool and this boosted her confidence even more. She was feeling stronger every day and made the decision that a family holiday was called for. She had been swimming a few times with the family and was now at ease with her appearance, and she needed to feel the sun on her skin and sand between her toes.

It was settled, and a family holiday in the sun was agreed upon and booked. Vera made sure she packed extra 'chicken fillets', as the prosthetics were now called by her and her friends at the breast clinic. She wanted to be able to change outfits relatively quickly and it was easier if the 'fillets' were already in place in a few garments. The holiday departure date came around quickly and the family was excited by everything, from the airport to reaching their hotel. Almost a whole week had passed and the family was happy and relaxed. Everyone had a lovely tan and had enjoyed every minute exploring new beaches and restaurants.

One morning during the second week, Vera was taking the grandchildren swimming at the local beach. The sun was shining but there was a little breeze, and the water wasn't quite as calm as it had been; it was now cresting in small waves. The children bounded around regardless, dipping in and out of the surf, pretending to be dolphins and sharks. They loved the added excitement of the waves and, being strong swimmers, Vera was happy to keep an eye on them while enjoying the waves picking her up and carrying her to the shore.

As she was swimming out to slightly deeper water, she noticed something glinting in the sunlight. There were a few people near her, and the children made their way out towards where she was treading water. Vera realised in a moment what the object was and knew she had to take drastic action. "Shark", she yelled at the top of her voice. Everyone looked momentarily in her direction and then headed quickly for the shore, shrieks of 'shark, shark' filling the air. The children were already squealing and making their way back in the direction they had just come from. In one quick movement Vera had grabbed the object and squeezed it back into the cup of her bathing suit.

She then quickly swam back to the shore laughing and apologising loudly to everyone on the beach for scaring them. Everyone's expressions changed, and soon all were laughing at the 'crazy English lady'. Vera apologised to her grandchildren who told her off with plenty of 'Oh, Gran, only you could think you had seen a shark!' Vera laughed off the teasing while discreetly adjusting her swimming costume.

On the way back to the hotel where the family were staying Vera found a supermarket; it had a stationery section and she found some superglue. When everyone was back in their rooms getting ready for dinner, Vera sat crossed legged in her bedroom glueing 'chicken fillets' into each of her bathing suits. She had no intentions of letting another 'shark' spoil her holiday.

Good For A Grin
AND OLYMPIC GOLD FOR BLADDER MANAGEMENT GOES TO…

If you are not thinking about your bum when being treated for rectal cancer, the likelihood is that you are thinking about your bladder. This was particularly the case for Pat. Having been told the tumour in his rectum needed radiotherapy to reduce it in size (although it would get larger initially, purely because it wouldn't like being zapped) before it could be removed surgically. However, it was important that the radiotherapy was directed very precisely, not only for maximum effectiveness, but also to make sure no other organs were affected.

In Pat's case, the bladder was the organ most likely to be affected if the radiotherapy 'zapping' wasn't exactly right. To control this eventuality, he had to gauge how full his bladder was at every session. The treatment was given in an oval, so getting the contour the same all the way around was paramount. If the bladder were too full, the stomach would be pushed out, making the contour around the middle bigger than at the back. Also, the bladder would be too close to the tumour, and this could then have further implications, including possible bladder problems after the treatment, something Pat definitely wanted to avoid.

Not being full enough didn't help with the procedure either, making it less effective, so guessing fluid intake became an obsession during the radiotherapy treatment. It was all about precision, precision, precision. Too empty meant having to drink a little water, wait ten minutes, get scanned then hopefully have the treatment. Too full was even trickier. Pat had to try to wee a little bit, have another scan and then try for the treatment again.

As everyone who has ever had to do it, weeing just a tiny little bit with a full bladder takes genius-level style concentration (an instant admission to Mensa should be awarded) and precision skill. Both these attributes had to be mastered. In time Pat became proficient to varying degrees, but the days when he didn't have the treatments were a joy, not to be consumed by the drinking…weeing…waiting …drinking…weeing…waiting cycle. These times actually felt like a holiday – not your palm tree-laced, secluded beach, exotic cocktails and balmy temperatures type of holiday, but a holiday nonetheless.

There were however the golden days. Not many, but some regardless, whereby the science – the 'Pat Science' – worked out perfectly and he got it right first time. These were the days when he walked in and bing! The scan showed he had got it absolutely right first time and the treatment went ahead. The challenge came after Pat had managed to attain the perfect score of two for two. Two sessions of radiotherapy had been given without any bladder adjustments. No extra drinking or weeing or waiting. A high five from the radiographer and much back slapping all round, Pat felt like a champion.

The challenge was on! Could he make it three for three?

The day dawned bright and breezy. The athlete went through his routine in his head. Drink a little, wait, wee a little… and repeat.. Arriving at the treatment centre he felt good, but then his instincts kicked in – was he a little full? Was his mind playing tricks on him? It was scan time…the tension was building…the crowd (Pat, radiographer and an assistant) fell into a hushed silence. The scan completed… the wait seemed endless…and then bing! The treatment could go ahead. Pat felt like he had won Gold. In his mind he was making the walk to the podium, stepping up to first position, accepting the medal and bouquet of flowers. Yes, Pat takes Olympic Gold in the great sport of bladder management.

After the treatment there was much celebrating and jubilation, a great day for all.

It's the little things.

Might Make You Smile
SHERRY LOVE, SHERRY.

Anita was the sort of woman who came up with an idea and ran with it. Whatever it took, as long as she truly believed in whatever it was, she had the sort of personality that wouldn't allow her to leave something on her mind alone. Some, usually those close to her, may have even described her as obsessive. However, any label given to Anita never bothered her a bit. She knew where she was heading, at least the desired end result anyway. How she got there was left to fate, destiny, and her own dogged determination to make things happen.

Working with people was her biggest passion. She chaired business networking groups, set up charity events (even in her own back garden), and had created a new cancer support group with a co-founder that had run another group previously. Anita secured a beautiful venue to hold the once-a-month meetings, a country hotel and golf club. Once the word had been put out, the response was fantastic; Anita was thrilled with the feedback from those who attended. The feeling of togetherness, empathy, and moral support oozed from the light and airy hotel drawing room where the group met.

Anita worked hard to make sure she had guest speakers, healthcare advisors, and various treatment providers on hand. The time flew by, and the group went from strength to strength. With great publicity, and an excellent reputation as a sanctuary for cancer sufferers, in no time the group was promoted in every hospital and doctor's waiting room. The distinctive purple and lime-green banners were also on community information notice boards everywhere.

In the spring of 2015, Anita noticed a spot – not a mole – a spot that didn't seem to want to go away. Being sensible, she went to the doctor to get it checked out. The doctor allayed her fears and stated that there was nothing to worry about. More time went by and still the spot wouldn't disappear, having a sort of sugary textured scab that never quite healed. She decided to get a second opinion. The confirmation came through, it was skin cancer – Squamous Cell Carcinoma.

The delivery of the news came on a calm, quiet sort of day; blue skies and a little warm sunshine. The devastation Anita heard ringing in her head and ears was, however, deafening. Anita found that she had an inability to hear what the consultant said next other than the single sentence containing the word 'cancer'. As she left the building and stepped out into the sunshine she knew one thing, she needed a drink; a drink to help with the shock. She knew the best drink for her was a sherry, a Tio Pepe to be exact. An old fashioned tipple, but one her grandmother was often heard saying, 'sherry for shock'.

The pub across the road from the hospital looked like the perfect answer. Her husband had softly mentioned that he understood she was ill, but it was getting on for dinner time. 'Blow dinner, blow the time of day, blow everything' she said to herself. She needed time to think and to try and digest what she had just been told. The news she had been given had lost all detail other than she had cancer.

Anita almost fell through the door, not noticing the raised door jam or the large sign above the door stating 'Mind the Step'. She was only saved by the grasp of her husband steadying her as he quickly steered her to a table in the corner before her legs buckled. Regaining some composure once seated, Anita's thoughts were interrupted by a very young waitress sporting purple hair, piercings in her nose, eyebrow, and at least twenty in both ears. The young girl shuffled nervously from one foot to the other, Anita wondered if she had picked up on the tension or if maybe her shoes were uncomfortable, but she didn't really care. She heard her husband order a pint for himself, his voice sounded as if in a dream; discernible but way off in the distance, almost like an echo. Her own mind was a deep, dense fog.

The young girl asked her twice what she would like to drink, Anita tried to get herself together and answered brightly, 'Tio Pepe sherry, a large one please.' The girl's face was a blank; there was again silence between the three people. Anita inexplicably felt a surge of annoyance. 'Sherry please, sherry.' She said loudly, as if bellowing might change the girl's expression. The waitress looked no different, the blank face just blinked at the space somewhere above Anita's head. Now was not a person who lost her temper readily, but she felt anger rising.

'What's that?' the purple-haired girl muttered. She was genuinely confused.

'Sherry, sherry, sherry,' she snapped incredulously. Anita could feel her husband's gaze burning into her from the left side, but she was unable to help herself. She had become helpless to stop herself from displaying her irritation.

In her mind's eye, she saw herself move in slow motion. She leapt up, kicked her chair back – kung fu style – and barged past the waitress, running towards the bar. Hitching up her skirt above her knees, and in a beautifully orchestrated movement that Starsky and Hutch would have been proud of, she launched herself onto the bar. Splayed along the length of the bar, she tilted her head towards the optics and leant back. The whisky, vodka, and gin bottles gleamed in the sunlight. Placing her head beneath the optics, she pressed the release for the vodka and allowed the liquid to fall directly into her mouth, taking great gulps. She could feel the burning liquid make its way through her body, and with its progress, her muscles relax.

In reality, Anita felt herself regain control, smile at the purple-haired girl, and allow her shoulders to relax. The waitress was standing in front of her, now looking bored and chewing on her pen, still awaiting a reply, but looking like she couldn't care less if it never came.

In a smooth, soothing voice Anita smiled and said, 'I'll have a large Pinot Grigio then.' From the corner of her eye, Anita could just make out her husband visibly lighten up and relax. Explosion averted, Anita smiled to herself, grandma's remedy could wait until they got home.

Good For A Grin
AVIARIES OR SHEEP?

Richard and Lorraine had set out on the leaflet drop, up and down pathways and driveways throughout the village. Neither of them minded the walking involved – the fresh air, along with being outdoors and together, was an enjoyable time. In fact, Richard loved pretty much anything active or sports-orientated. If he wasn't walking, cycling, playing cricket, tennis or rugby, to name but a few of his sporting endeavours, then there was definitely something up. Either that or he was taking part in the local Dwyle Flunking competition (a game of two teams, twelve men on each, taking turns to dance around while being slapped by the other team with a beer-soaked cloth, the 'Dwyle'. The result is always contested, and vast amounts of beer consumed.)

It was this aspect of his life that made the recurring gout episodes so very annoying and supremely frustrating. Every now and then he would experience an aggressive flare-up that rendered him immobile. Not a situation someone like Richard appreciated, one little bit. Nor for that matter did Lorraine – a man like Richard was not happy being confined.

It didn't seem to matter what the doctors gave him, even 'horse strength' antibiotics made no difference. So much so that matters were getting worse. Richard became completely confined to the house and then ultimately bedbound, unable to get around at all. It was only when he finally had a blood test performed that acute myeloid leukaemia, not gout, was diagnosed – and it was advanced.

Richard was offered the choice of two clinical trials at Addenbrooke's Hospital in Cambridge, not too far from where they lived. One trial was low risk, though with fewer possible benefits, while the other was much higher risk but with the possibility of far greater rewards, should it work. Lorraine and Richard were expecting a new grandchild around this time, and their family was everything to them both.

Richard was a man who had always aimed high and had strong principles that he lived by, sometimes with interesting outcomes. Occasionally, it had to be said, living by his principles could cause a certain degree of chaos. His past antics included the time he and the late activist John Bugg drove a tank to central London out of protest (for which he was arrested), not to mention the time he cut the wire at RAF Molesworth (for which he was also arrested!). Yes, it was fair to say Richard had always been a risk taker, but he was a man who believed in doing something if you felt strongly enough about it. There was no doubt the high-risk trial was for him, and there was no hesitation whatsoever in his decision.

One thing, however, that had Richard and Lorraine perplexed in the midst of this new information, future prospects, enormous decisions to be made and the knowledge of the likelihood for Richards survival, was when they were asked the question: "Has Richard been around aviaries or sheep?" Stunned, the couple were thrown into a state of bewilderment. Neither could recall anything of the kind. No, they had no plans to open a petting zoo of any description. They hadn't even visited any zoos or farms, although they did live in the countryside, in a village. In the blur of all that had gone on, neither thought to ask why? What significance could this possibly have?

During the darkest times it was this question that made them smile – a bewildered, questioning and perplexing smile, but a smile nonetheless. They never did find out the relevance, but did enjoy pondering the question.

Might Make You Smile
DRIP, DRIP, DRIP.

Maggie had decided that she would make the most of a good day. When she considered 'the most' of a day now, in comparison to the hectic pace of what was her previous life, it entailed a single trip to the local supermarket. Even getting herself ready was a snail-paced affair, but Maggie was now accustomed to it. She had learnt to listen to her body and its energy levels and act accordingly.

With her headscarf wrapped bandana style and make-up applied, Maggie was ready to go. Sam, her pug dog, looked up at her hopefully. 'Not just yet Sam, maybe later though.' Maggie smiled lovingly at his little hopeful expression. Even Sam had adjusted to this new life of sporadic short walks, plenty of relaxing and the very occasional outing. It was a little different to the adventures that Maggie and Sam had in the past. Hikes up Snowdonia with Sam spending a little time in Maggie's rucksack, head poking out from the top enjoying the fresh bracing air. He only had short legs after all, and he did so enjoy the comfort of the warm fleece wrap. There were long walks along beaches in Norfolk with the surf touching his toes, and Maggie throwing stones for him to bring back and lay at her feet.

Sam had watched his mistress shed so many tears for such a long time, but she had always smiled when he had attempted to lick them away. He knew how to cheer her up and was happy to be there for his best friend. Sam returned to his cosy basket surrounded by his soft toys; he could wait for a walk. He watched Maggie gather up her keys and close the door behind her. Another nap was the perfect pastime until Maggie returned.

The sun was shining, and Maggie was enjoying the feeling of warmth on her face. She couldn't help but smile; today was definitely a good day. Birds were singing their songs in the hedges and the trees she passed on the short walk to the shops. Maggie felt her nose twitching; she had suffered from hayfever in the past, but since the chemotherapy she had been symptom-free. She was guessing the treatment had pretty much killed off any other mildly irritating condition in its wake. The twitching got worse, she felt like a hyperactive rabbit, her nose seemed to have a will of its own.

Inside the supermarket, Maggie hoped the twitching would stop. Her attention diverted for the moment, she chose some fruit; plums, apples, a coconut, blueberries, and strawberries. With these in her basket she headed over to the salad section. It was early, and the supermarket was fairly quiet. The lettuce she picked up looked like it might have already been washed; there being a couple of small droplets on its bright green, shiny leaves. When she leant forward to choose a cucumber, there were a couple of droplets on it too. Maggie looked towards the ceiling of the supermarket, wondering if there was a leak or a faulty air conditioning vent, but there was nothing. Wiping away the moisture from the items, she continued around the various displays.

It wasn't long before Maggie began to slow down and she knew her energy levels were lowering, so she made her way to the checkout. The half dozen items she had were not heavy, and she was looking forward to the gentle walk home; happy with herself and her efforts.

Suddenly there was another drip on her hand, a great sploshing one this time. Again she looked up to see where this mysterious liquid was coming from, it was almost as if it were following her around the supermarket. Tilting her head backwards and looking up, she tasted something on her top lip.

It was then that Maggie knew it was her nose that had been running the whole time. All the way around the supermarket her nose had been dripping like a leaky tap. In a panic, she patted herself down but could not find a single tissue; her face was burning with embarrassment. With her hand over the lower part of her face, she apologised profusely to the lady at the till, 'I'm so sorry, I don't have a single tissue.' The lady smiled at her and produced a packet of tissues from under the counter. 'They tell you you'll lose the hair from your head, but don't always mention anywhere else. And when do we ever think about nose hair?', she laughed. It was only then that Maggie noticed the lady was sporting a navy headscarf, it matched her uniform perfectly. Maggie was so used to seeing people around her with various forms of head gear and wigs that she hadn't even acknowledged the cashier's own.

Maggie took a couple of tissues and laughed out loud at how much her nose had been running. 'Just be grateful you don't have a cold', laughed the lady at the till, 'the last time I had one, I had to stay indoors for a week.' She said, chuckling. Maggie giggled to herself all the way home. She wondered how keen Sam would have been to lick her face today.

Good For A Grin
THE COLOURS OF THE RAINBOW

It is amazing the effect that the various drugs used in the treatment and diagnosis of cancer have on everyday bodily functions. There is one in particular that is readily affected and easily measured, and that is urinating.

Who knew that even a scan can produce some interesting effects. You may find that as soon as you go to the toilet after a P.E.T. scan you could be weeing a blue colour. Somewhat disconcerting, yes. A little fascinating, certainly.

Couple this with the patient who is taking a good dose of multi-vitamin (if you are having difficulty eating, often a side effect of chemotherapy and radiotherapy, this may be suggested), which are likely to turn your wee fluorescent yellow or green. A hue that Sigourney Weaver in any scene from Alien would be not be surprised at encountering.

Doxorubicin, given in chemotherapy, will, apart from doing exactly what it is supposed to, will often turn your wee a delightful crimson colour. Obviously this can be pretty scary if you haven't been warned and are possibly a little sensitive about what is happening to you anyway. This has been likened to peeing Ribena, and while it's most definitely somewhat more toxic and not to be considered as thirst quenching, it's an interesting analogy nonetheless.

All these things can make for an interesting experience should you find yourself in communal urinals. Still, it could prove to be a fascinating topic of conversation, depending on your audience.

Might Make You Smile
IS IT A BIRD? IS IT A PLANE?

Suzy found her diagnosis of breast cancer to be a huge inconvenience, almost as much as a worrying shock. She was a practical woman; a successful businesswoman with a busy PR practice in London. She lived in the home counties in a quiet village, which allowed her an escape from London's busy hustle and bustle. Her home was a handsome four bedroom detached mock Tudor affair, with an easy to maintain garden and smart paved driveway.

Finding the small, pea-sized lump in her left breast brought with it irritation and an overwhelming sense of annoyance. She simply didn't have the time for this. The consultant was swift to confirm her fears; scans showed she had discovered her lump early, and her treatment would be a lumpectomy followed by chemotherapy. The side effects of the chemotherapy were explained, and dates were booked for treatment to commence.

With a bit of juggling and the hiring of some extra staff, Suzy felt as organised with a treatment schedule and how her life would proceed afterwards as, she guessed, could be possible. She explained in a matter-of-fact-manner about her diagnosis to her staff; feeling she owed it to them to both put them in the picture and at ease with the new arrangements. She was touched by their response, and felt that when she was well again, she would perhaps spend a little more time with them all on a more social level. She knew she was often aloof and could be standoffish from time to time.

The treatments went well, but Suzy was amazed at how quickly the side effects took their toll, she was completely bald in a very short period of time. To cheer herself up she bought a very stylish and expensive wig. It looked fabulous, she was pleased with the result, and was beginning to feel a little more like her usual self. Suzy also found she was having to learn to take herself a little less seriously; to laugh at herself from time to time, and to see the funnier side of life.

This was never more apparent than on the occasion she was having her chemotherapy and needed to go to the toilet. The larger disabled toilet was occupied and she had to take her dispenser, which was much taller than her and had four wheels which appeared to roll in any direction other than the way you wanted, into the standard sized toilet. Trying to manoeuvre herself, the wheelie thing, and remove her lower body garments simultaneously, she quickly realised she had almost contorted herself into a granny knot. Having then caught her reflection in the mirror positioned over what was possibly the smallest hand basin known to man, she couldn't help but laugh. She resembled a badly wrapped, oversized parcel with an I.V. line criss-crossing over her face, and for whatever reason, she now had an arm suspended in the air over her head, giving the appearance of a somewhat worse-for-wear marionette. At this point she was laughing loudly at herself as she managed to shuffle towards the toilet door and slide the lock, allowing the door to fall open just a crack.

It was her raucous laughter that caught the attention of one of the ward nurses. Although it was obvious she required assistance, she was unable to explain anything through her laughter. The nurse saw immediately what had happened and a full ten minutes later Suzy had been unravelled, repositioned in the disabled toilet, and was able to sort herself out.

Suzy felt capable of returning to work after a time. She craved the buzz of the office and the business's demanding clients. In typical fashion, the morning of her return to work she slept through her alarms. Rushing to catch the train at the station nearby, she quickly applied her make-up and newly acquired wig. Pleased with her appearance, she jumped in a taxi; not wanting to tire herself out by the walk to the station.

The train arrived within a couple of minutes of purchasing her return ticket. The wind had picked up, and Suzy was glad of the warmth of the already full carriage. She stood for part of the journey before a seat became available at Tottenham Hale.

As it passed through a tunnel, Suzy marvelled at how different the person looking back at her from the reflection in the train window was now. After ten minutes, Liverpool Street Station came into view. Suzy was both excited and nervous to return to her office. The PR firm had taken years to build up, and she was proud of her accomplishments. Now she felt more proud of herself than ever. In her eyes, her cancer had been removed, and she was now 'recovering from having cancer', not someone who was 'suffering with cancer'.

As she stepped out of Liverpool Street Station and onto the wide pavement, the wind was gusting through the narrow streets. Suddenly, Suzy's head was cold, really cold; she knew straightaway what had happened. At that exact moment, she heard a shriek behind her. Turning, she saw a small man in a business suit, arms flailing wildly, looking for all the world like he was trying to wrestle some sort of furry creature. She couldn't make out if it was a small cat or dog. It was blonde in colour, and slightly circular in shape. The man was squealing in a high-pitched voice, very clearly disturbed by the unprovoked attack. The animal looked like it was stuck to him, attacking him. Suzy quickly identified the animal.

Straightening her skirt, adjusting her suit jacket, and with her head held high, she headed over to the man. She snatched the furry object from him, patted it down neatly, and then pulled it onto her head; hoping against hope she had at least placed it on the right way round. Then she stalked off, in what she prayed was a confident and purposeful manner, in the direction of her office.

By the time the lift reached Bryce Public Relations, Suzy was once more laughing to herself and made a mental note to always carry extra double-sided toupe tape. It was an interesting start to her first day back at work.

Good For A Grin
AND THE VOTES ARE IN

With the diagnosis of prostate cancer in, there was now the issue of treatment options for Michael. He and his wife were a team, and a good team at that. Michael was given the choices of radiotherapy or radical prostatectomy. In Mike's mind the words curable and cancer did not go together, but that was exactly what he had – 'curable cancer'. When Michael had questions, fears and concerns it was his wife's calming, stabilising response that kept him going. "We will just have to see, we should get more information when we next see the consultant," she would say, holding her hand out towards him, should he wish to take it in his.

It wasn't a case of dismissing the concern but, stabilising the situation with calm logic, and Ann's own way of showing her support. Mike and Ann decided they would take all the information on both procedures and each would read one lot one evening (not your usual bedtime reading, it had to be said) and then the next evening they would swap. They would leave it twenty-four hours and then there would be a secret ballot when they were both absolutely sure of what both procedures entailed.

It was after they had collected all the information on both procedures that a place called 'Maggie's Wallace', or Maggie's' as it was commonly known, was suggested as a great place to get support, meet others in the same position and where counsellors were available to discuss any aspect of cancer with you. It was to prove invaluable, a comfortable place, full of warmth, information and understanding. As well as tea, coffee, cake and fruit, it was ran by qualified staff and a wonderful collection of volunteers. It was there that Michael and Ann discovered a six-session course on radical prostatectomy. There were also sessions covering diet, relaxation, yoga and tai chi.

Over the two nights Michael and Ann read the reams of information. Michael even created a spreadsheet as he realised there were so many points to consider. As he added up all pros and cons he deduced his choice would be prostatectomy.

The votes were placed. Mike unfolded both pieces of paper. They had each voted for Prostatectomy. They laughed – democracy at its best.

Might Make You Smile
CATCH THAT!

Amy had completed the whole treatment for her latest visit from the cancer monster, this was how she liked to refer to the recurrence of the disease. She had been unfortunate in having cancer strike in various parts of her body over the years, including bladder, kidney, and the latest was breast. She felt that she was now a bit of an old hand at taking on the necessary treatments, she had tried most of them at least once.

For her breast cancer she had a double mastectomy, she had no intention of taking any chances and it was agreed upon without hesitation. She had decided not to have any reconstructive surgery for the time being, and wore prosthetic implants in her underwear. Amy was simply grateful to be given another chance.

Two years on, and Amy's lust for life was as evident as ever. She and her husband were regulars at the local gym, enjoyed going out for evenings dancing, and there wasn't a party that she didn't get an invite to. Amy made it her mission to make the very most of every day, even when she wasn't always feeling one hundred percent. When a close friend and her husband suggested a holiday in Spain, Amy jumped at the idea. A villa was booked, along with flights, and a hire car; Amy couldn't wait.

Shopping for clothes was already a passion for Amy, but with a holiday to shop for she took shopping to a whole new level. Her husband despaired as to how much luggage they were going to have to take, but took it all in good humour. He loved seeing his wife getting so much pleasure out of life and he knew they were going to have a great time. Having been friends with the couple for many years, the foursome were completely comfortable in each other's company, all being of similar ages; and though Amy had never had children, her friend Susie's were all grown up and had families of their own. Already close, the foursome had grown even closer throughout Amy's treatments.

On the morning of the departure, the four were enjoying breakfast before heading out to the airport. Amy had made sure all her medication was correctly labelled, document supported, and in all the required measures. When everyone was ready they headed off to the airport, which wasn't too far away. The journey took only twenty minutes in a taxi, and the group were deposited at the terminal building. Amy couldn't hide her excitement about going on holiday. They had always had short breaks away, but with all the treatments Amy had endured, they had never been able to get anything more than a few days here and there. For years they had always been in the U.K., as she wasn't fit enough to travel any greater distance. Having been given the go ahead by her doctors, this was to be the first trip abroad in over ten years. For Amy it felt like the very first time, and she was determined to make the most of every minute.

The group arrived a little early for their flight and decided a celebratory drink would be a great way to start the holiday. A bottle of champagne was ordered for the ladies and ice-cold beer for the men. It was only just past noon, but they all agreed they had more reason than ever to celebrate. In no time their flight was called and the happy foursome were on their way.

Landing in the brilliant sunshine and feeling its warmth instantly made Amy feel better than ever. She had no plans for the days to come other than simply enjoy her time with the like-minded people she loved.

Days were spent lounging around the pool, sunning herself like the native lizards, swimming, and enjoying as much of the Spanish experience as possible. Amy was determined to make the very most of every moment. She loved the feel of the sun on her skin.

She sampled as much of the local delicacies as possible; from baked baby clams to delicious suckling pig. The couples enjoyed trips to the coast, vineyards, cheese making farms, and tried at least one different restaurant or tapas bar a day.

Amy tried to make sure she got as much rest as possible in between activities, but her lust for life was boundless. The group joked that it was her, out of the four, who had the most energy anyway; and they were all quite glad when she decided she needed a rest and would take herself off to the cool of the villa for a nap.

It was while they were out shopping in the nearest mall, with its amazing collection of shops and boutiques, that Amy picked up a leaflet for the Aquavelis Water Park in nearby Torre Del Mar. That was it, that was going to be Amy's next conquest; her husband and friends thought she was completely mad. 'Don't you think we are just a teensy bit past it?' laughed Josh, Amy's husband. 'We'll be the oldest ones there', laughed her friend Susie. 'I need to do it, you all said this was a trip of discovery and recovery, and for my next discovery I would like to hurtle down a slide, screaming like a banshee,' she laughed. It was settled, the next day would be "water park day". Amy fell asleep smiling to herself that night, like a child, she couldn't wait for the following day to come.

The water park was busy with large family groups, teenagers hanging around in groups trying their best to look cool and unaffected by each other's presence. Amy felt the same surge of excitement she had felt as a child when visiting fairgrounds or the anticipation leading up to Christmas. Her heart was pounding as the four made their way to the top of the first slide. The men went first, claiming they wanted to be at the bottom to catch their spouses when it was their turn to come down the slide. In reality, the two men had reverted to their own childhoods and were keen to take the plunge down the slide.

The water was pumping down the length of the brightly coloured tubes keeping the riders moving at break-neck speed along the slippery surface. In a moment, both men had disappeared into the darkness of the first hairpin bend. Amy and Susie readied themselves at the top of the slide, waiting for the go-ahead from the lifeguards to launch themselves down the ride. On the count of three the two friends jettisoned themselves down the slide to the first bend. Amy was squealing with delight as she hurtled past others, who were now queuing up the steep hill to take the ride. She guessed it must have been quite a sight seeing a middle aged woman sporting a psychedelic bikini zipping past at lightning speed, making more noise than anybody else.

As Amy approached the final bend she felt the water surge behind her, and laughed out loud at the sheer exhileration she felt at being weightless, as she became airborne at the end of the slide. As she was mid-air something caught her eye for a split second, it was opaque with a silvery sheen to it in the sunlight. As quick as she saw it, it was gone. She heard a familiar voice yell, 'catch that!', as she plunged into the pool at the bottom of the slide.

At the moment she found her feet in the plunge pool, she was joined by her laughing friends and husband. In one smooth discreet motion Marcus, Susie's husband, had pinged Amy's bikini strap and plopped something in the cup. 'You'll be missing that', he laughed. Amy thought she may collapse, laughing as the other three regaled the story of the middle-aged woman bombing down the slide, arms and legs all over the place, a false breast flying high into the air, and being beautifully caught by a man with a look of concentration on his face worthy of any fielder participating in an England versus Australia cricket match at Lords.

Good For A Grin
CECIL

Rectal cancer had meant life-saving surgery, and further treatment in the form of chemotherapy and radiotherapy was going to feature heavily in Patrick's life.

First things first, surgery was required. Pat was going to have to join the ranks of the 'ostomates society' (no secret handshakes here just the addition of a little extra luggage). He would need to have a colostomy bag, and for this to happen he was going to require surgery to create a stoma. Obviously, this surgery is life altering in itself, both physically and psychologically. As Pat says, he still poos, just differently. He was quick to realise the need to try to remove the stigma associated with poo and bums, particularly among men, who often don't always talk about things, especially these types of private matters.

To help with this, Patrick started a blog on day one of his actual diagnosis. He wanted to offer as much down-to-earth support, facts and openness to anybody who chose to listen (or in this case, read). He was honest and upfront from the start that there would indeed be toilet talk on all levels, be it poo, bums or farts. Pat wanted it all to be out there in the open. Embarrassment or shying away was not an option.

When the day came for the operation, Patrick had researched as much as possible about his surgery and it was suggested the stoma be named, something to do with helping get around the life-changing event mentally.

On September 14th 2016 Cecil was welcomed into the Reeve household. Pat had no idea why he chose the name Cecil, but it seemed to appeal and stuck immediately. Overnight Cecil became an internet star, featuring heavily in the blog and, as with any newborn, life predominantly now evolved around him.

Might Make You Smile
GROUNDHOG DAY RADIO

Jan was not looking forward to the next six weeks. She was due radiotherapy every day including weekends. The dose had been explained to her as being gradually increased but she was under no illusion, she would soon become very ill.

The treatment started on a Monday, and her husband drove the well-rehearsed route to Addenbrooke's Hospital in Cambridge. The couple tried to make light of the situation; how long they would be repeating the journey, how many miles they would clock up, how many stairs they would climb, cups of tea they would drink, how many times the same questions would be asked verifying name, date of birth etc., before the radio would be administered.

By the end of the first week, Jan was getting the routine pat down. She had made friends with others undergoing the same treatment schedule and others who were on different regimes, but all with the same goal, to beat cancer. Jan also knew her nurse's names, and by the end of the second week she had memorised their shift schedules, knew about their families, how old their children were, and where they had gone or were going on holiday.

Jan began to feel the effects of her treatment, and she started to feel unwell, but continued with the schedule knowing it would get worse before she got better; the hours, days, and weeks began to blur for both Jan and her husband. The trips to the hospital were marked with the passing of the same landmarks each and every day. The drive was made almost on auto-pilot. She visited the same room, the same chair, and looked out of the same window.

The routine reminded her of a film she had once watched called Groundhog Day, where the day restarted the same every single day; with the same events, conversations, and interactions. Jan felt she was actually living that film plot, just a different scenario.

One morning, Jan was stopped as she was leaving the treatment suite. The receptionist asked, as she did from time, to time when Jan's next session was. The answer was always the same: same time, same place the following day.

The receptionist checked her appointment book, flipping pages back and forth. A smile spread across her face. 'Nope Jan, actually, you have no more appointments, that's it! Your treatments have finished.' Her smile stretched from ear-to-ear.

Jan felt her body relax and she beamed back at the lady behind the desk. 'That's it? I'm done? I'm really done?' Jan was delighted, exhausted, but delighted. She spent a few minutes saying goodbye to all the staff, patients, and the friends she had shared six weeks of her life with. She didn't expect to feel so emotional and was caught off guard by the love and affection shown by everyone. Jan's husband had been under the same illusion as Jan, and he was equally delighted to learn his wife's treatments had come to an end. Their own personal 'Groundhog Day' had finally stopped. The drive home that day was filled with laughter, relief and renewed hope for the future.

Good For A Grin
ONE TESTICLE OR TWO?...

"Your friends will always be there with you through thick and thin"

Dan had the diagnosis confirmed to him, he had testicular cancer.

Telling everyone was the hardest bit, once he and his wife Nat had got over the initial shock.

With rugby mates, doing this over beer and a curry was the only way forward. Dan, however, didn't gauge his audience very well and began before everybody had arrived, meaning he ended up telling the tale three times over. It took less than five minutes before someone started taking the piss. Cheers, fellas!

Mates being mates, they responded in the only way they knew how. More beer and an in-depth discussion on the offending nut and its possible replacement.

There then followed a debate that would rival a UN convention on the probabilities of getting a really big replacement. Can you request a specific size and weight? Could you get an extra two – just how impressive would that be? Was it possible to acquire a titanium one? The grown-up, educated drinkers discussed all possible scenarios long into the night. Everyone was a dedicated expert. Dan found the evening both comforting and highly educational (well, not really the last bit).

The hangover the next day was so worth it. The world was back to relative normality, life carries on. When the pros and cons were discussed, Dan decided the prosthetic route was not for him: there would be no replacement.

Might Make You Smile
BACK TO FRONT, TOP TO BOTTOM

Fi was amazed at just how much her body had changed. At first she was saddened, so much so, that she thought she might seek some support to help her through her feelings. It was only when she went to a local support group that she found others experiencing the same emotions, and she gained renewed strength and perspective, and became more accepting of her body and all it had been through.

Fi had undergone a procedure, an LD operation, where a section of flesh and muscle from her back was used to create a new breast. When the surgery was completed, Fi was pleased with the results and would comment that she was now "back-to-front". She would happily accredit it for anything, from forgetfulness to unexplained bouts of retail therapy (which often resulted in her returning unwanted items, which then facilitated another wander around the shops). If she was getting cross she would yell, 'you're getting right on my back'. This was her polite way of actually saying, 'you're getting right on my tit'; and those who knew her well, knew exactly what she meant. Fi laughed along with everyone, enjoying the double meaning.

She enjoyed sharing stories of talented surgeons creating body enhancements from various other body parts. One of Fi's favourites was one lady's recollection of her breast being created from a section of her midriff. It was only when the lady in question's hair began to grow back, that she experienced hair growth in some odd places and the hairs that grew in the 'odd' places; were short, coarse, and bore no resemblance to the soft downy re-growth on her head. Feeling she needed to see someone about the hair, she made an appointment to see her consultant fearing her hormones may have created another issue other than cancer.

It was only on the morning of her appointment while in the shower that she burst out laughing and couldn't stop. The scar on her abdomen explained everything she needed to know; the hair would have been completely natural in the location of her scar. Toweling herself dry, she went to the phone and dialled the number for her consultant to cancel the appointment. As she hung up the receiver a quote popped into her head, 'Where'er you be let the hair grow free'. When she next went to her group meeting and spoke to her Macmillan nurse, she took great pleasure in regaling them of her discovery. As it turned out, as is so often the case, she was not the only patient to have discovered hair in strange and unusual places.

Good For A Grin
IS NORMAL, NORMAL?

Dave was almost halfway through the first cycle of treatment after having a testicle removed, but was still feeling okay. And this puzzled him.

He checked with his medical team, and they were delighted with his progress. In the end, Dave began to realise that the best way for him to cope with his position was to almost expect to feel unwell, expect to wake up feeling the dreaded possible side effects of chemo that he had heard and researched about (Google is not always a good thing to have instant access to).

If he took this approach, whenever he woke up and felt fine he was euphoric, feeling a new zest for life, a freedom, sound in the knowledge that he was blessed. This really helped him through his days.

He knew it might not last forever, but was grateful for every minute he remained feeling 'normal'; it could, after all, change at any moment.

Until that happened, Dave made the very most of his wellbeing. Lunch with his wife, a few cheeky (off-cycle) beer days with mates, enjoying his rugby (watching, not playing, those days would come in the future), reappreciating all the good things in life.

Having always been a great lover of life, this new dimension just enhanced his appreciation all the more, especially if he could enjoy those days with family and friends.

Might Make You Smile
DOUBLE UP DOLLY

Dolly was on a downer; she had been feeling ill from the side effects of her chemotherapy for so long, it had almost overtaken the fact that she had been diagnosed with breast cancer. She hadn't had a single symptom and the detection had been made on a purely routine mammogram. The cancer was now gone, it had been cut out, it was no longer there, and yet she felt so wretched. A double mastectomy had taken care of the tumour and any possibility of another, and she was eternally grateful.

Though none of this took away the fact that she was feeling so poorly. It was exhausting to be sick all the time; feeling too exhausted to be bothered with anything or anyone. Her throat was so sore, that even if she wanted to she could barely get anything down. Dolly was tired of not feeling like her normal self and it was getting her down.

The morning started out like any other, slowly. Dolly had to talk herself into getting out of bed. She could have quite easily laid in bed all day, but she knew that was a slippery slope and ultimately did her no good, other than make her all the more depressed. It was at this point, wallowing in her mood, that Dolly noticed something she hadn't seen in what seemed like an age. On the bedroom floor was a bright shaft of light stretching from one side of the room to the other.

The shaft of light originated from the side of the blind at the bedroom window. Dolly could not believe it was true? Slowly, she pulled back the duvet and placed her feet on the floor. Walking towards the window the carpet was feeling warm under her feet. As she lifted the blind, she was delighted to see she had guessed right. It was a beautiful sunny morning, bright blue sky, not a cloud, and Dolly stood enjoying the warmth of the sunlight streaming in. She couldn't help but be comforted and her mood lifted.

After standing for a considerable time listening to the birds singing and watching a tractor in the far field behind her house, Dolly formulated a plan. She was not going to let today go to waste; she was going to be as cheerful as possible. Flinging open the door of her wardrobe she chose a floral dress in bright colours, shoes, and accessories. Checking the calendar, she saw it was a Brafternoon Ladies Day, and she had never intended on going. Now she changed her mind, she would go, she would meet people, and she would do her damnedest to enjoy herself. She chose her prettiest underwear, and it was as she was dressing that she chuckled to herself. She was going to have a little fun.

Being out in the sunshine, feeling its warmth, and the brightness making trees, grass, and flowers look almost neon in their brilliance of colour. Every living thing looked as if it were illuminated from within. Every now and then Dolly would catch a glimpse of her reflection and smile to herself, today was a special day, Dolly could feel it.

The drawing room at the country hotel where the Brafternoon group met was buzzing. The sunshine had brought out more attendees than Dolly had ever seen. The scene looked like a garden party with the French doors flung wide open onto the sun terrace and gardens. Large umbrellas were dotted about offering just enough shade.

As Dolly walked in, Anita, the hostess did a double take. Dolly smiled brightly at her. 'Goodness Dolly, you look fabulous.' Dolly made her way over to Anita, then pulled her to a quiet part of the room. Checking that no one was looking, Dolly pulled the strap of her dress to one side allowing Anita to see a glimpse of bra and revealing her secret accessories. Tucked into the bra was her prosthetic breast, but Dolly had made a little adjustment to her look.

Today Dolly had doubled up on her implants. She was, for today, Brafternoon's very own Dolly Parton. 'Thought I'd cheer myself up' she laughed as she proudly sauntered off to join the others getting drinks and making their way to the gardens.

Good For A Grin
WHEREVER YOU BE
LET THE WIND BLOW FREE

It is fair to say that the list of possible side effects from the treatments involved in dealing with all forms of cancers goes on and on. It is, however, very much a game of Russian Roulette as to who gets what, if any.

Some effects can be debilitating, but there is one that can only really be viewed with humour. The sort of schoolyard humour of old that makes you belly laugh, which, by the way, makes it all the worse.

This side effect is chronic flatulence. It is not, by any means, the sneaky little squeaky fart that you can hide with a cough, door slam or clap. It has, in fact, been described as the mother of all noises.

In Peter's case it got to the point where every step he took was accompanied by the loudest trumpet. Birds flew from their perches in trees, outside, dogs ran to hide under the beds, neighbours two doors away were able to hear the crystal-clear parping. Peter could not help but laugh and laugh. This resulted in a fanfare that went something along the lines of laugh.. fart… laugh… fart louder… laugh… fart loudest!

Peter began to fear he may just blow away with the expelled gases and held on to every chair back, door handle and table top as he walked around the house. But one thing was for sure, there was absolutely no way he was going outside. No, this was a little something that had to be endured within the privacy of one's own home. There was the elderly, the very young and the infirm members of the public to consider, after all.

The tuneful day finally came to an end. Peter had laughed almost until he cried and as he drifted off to sleep he wondered whether he could have actually created a tune. Maybe tomorrow, a little experiment… should the situation remain.

Might Make You Smile
HAIR THERE, REALLY?

Mel had been distraught when her hair fell out in great clumps, not long after she started her cancer treatment.

Try as she might she couldn't stop the inevitable. She looked up every suggested lotion, potion and cold cap method but nothing worked for her. When her treatment had finished, ironically, it was waiting for her hair to reappear that became all-consuming. When the delicate fuzz of regrowth made its much longed for appearance she was ecstatic. Her friends and family rejoiced in her return to her old, upbeat self.

Every morning Mel would gently wash the soft downy hair. Before her diagnosis of cancer Mel had warm brown hair but she could already see the new hair was coming through blonde. She had always toyed with having a change of colour and it looked like nature had taken the decision for her.

Mel waited patiently for her hair to grow. Like anything truly longed for the waiting seemed to take an eternity. When her hair was about an inch long all over and she looked less bald and more 'cropped' Mel decided to leave her hat at home and venture out with dramatic earrings or a vibrant scarf, she was proud of her new hair and happy to show it off, everyday feeling stronger and a little more like her old self.

One day Mel was at the bathroom sink marvelling at the now gentle, golden waves all over her head, her hair was still short but she loved it. As the sunlight streamed through the bathroom window filling the room with almost white light Mel noticed something fluttering on the side of her face. It disappeared, and then as a breeze rose from the small open window to her left she saw it again.

It was a single, fine, long hair, about three inches long. Mel swiped at it thinking it was a loose hair having attached itself probably to a piece of clothing or a towel. It didn't budge, as she made a definitive grab for it she realised, in horror, it was in fact attached to her, not only to her, but to her chin!

Yes, the one place where her hair had grown super fast was the last place she had wanted it or even thought was possible.

Even though she was mortified by her discovery, she had to laugh; she was actually quite proud of the hair, it was a thread of hope that her hair would grow back fully.

Plucking the wayward hair Mel carefully wrapped it in a tissue and put it in her bedside drawer, still chuckling to herself she could wait to regale the story. Checking her appearance once more she left her home for work. She was careful to check regularly, in case there were any more stray hair poking from ears or worse still her nose, laughing to herself every time she did so.

Good For A Grin

IRRIGATION...
IRRIGATION...
IRRIGATION...
THAT'S WHAT YOU NEED

Warning: Poo Content

Pat had been considering the 'irrigation' process for quite a while, conducting a great deal of research and spending a lot of time looking into the procedure and its possible benefits.

Although Cecil the stoma was generally behaving well, Pat was always on the lookout for any way to make both their lives easier. The less Cecil had to work the less Pat had to concern himself with him. No offence, Cecil.

The decision was made: Cecil and Pat were going to take their relationship to the next level.

The Irrigation Team were called in.

Okay, now imagine trying to poo with an audience. Yep, even with the team's professional guidance and input, it was a little surreal and an unusual experience, to say the least. No standing ovations or scorecards though.

So, here is how it works. Don your lab coat, safety goggles on and pens at the ready. Using a cone that fits into the stoma (stoma nurses demonstrated how to do this), makes for an interesting afternoon with, believe it or not, much laughter.

After feeding in about 1.5 litres of tepid water, the pressure around the stoma is such that the cone can be removed. A long plastic sleeve, which becomes a sort of tube, goes over the stoma and into the toilet bowl. Once the process got going, things were moving along and it was clearly going well.

There were plenty of gasps and 'That's the best one we've done yet', which was all very encouraging. Pat felt the day was considered momentous and could easily imagine it worthy of a mention around the nurses' dinner table that evening.

The process can take about forty minutes to one hour, but it means that afterwards a stoma cap can be worn rather than a bag. This allows for more fitted clothing, with no need for larger tee shirts. It also means a 'once a day' visit to the toilet and less likelihood of 'incidents'. Almost a 'normal' bum again.

Some find irrigation is only a once every other day occurance, or even up to three days (although that's possibly considered a little Russian Roulette on the stoma front).

Although irrigation isn't for everyone, it does work for many. All anyone wants is to make life a little easier for themselves.

Might Make You Smile
KNITTING, NOT SUCH AN INNOCENT HOBBY

With so much sitting around in Chemotherapy, new hobbies can often be taken up, something to while away the hours the treatments can take. This was definitely the case for Margaret's group, and knitting was the chosen 'in thing'. The crowd who shared her chemotherapy session were a sassy bunch who loved a good laugh at just about anything. They would banter with the nursing staff, and try their very best to make the most of their time spent together.

There were a few male nurses on the ward, and they were always good sports with whatever was going on. The chemotherapy sessions were almost looked forward to, not by any means the treatment aspect, but certainly the company and camaraderie within the group.

The patients had been knitting for some time; there were always balls of coloured yarn dangling from chairs or spilling out of knitting bags. The gentle clickity-click sound of knitting needles succumbed to busy fingers. Everyone was looking forward to showing off the fruits of their labour.

When the time finally came to show their wares, everyone was looking forward with great anticipation. There was a buzz about the group; were there going to be multi-coloured blankets, baby booties, hats, gloves, and scarves? Everybody was keeping things very much to themselves.

It was a good thing the male nurses were such good fun and happy to share a joke, as when all the knitted items were revealed one patient had very carefully, and very kindly knitted Willie Warmers. Suffice to say, nobody could top this for entertainment value alone. The laughter could be heard throughout the unit. It is safe to say it pays to have a good sense of humour when dealing with cancer patients and carers.

No nurses were harmed or offended in the making or regaling of this story, I am reliably informed.

Good For A Grin
NO FOOLS AND XBOX RULES DAY

April 1st.

With a chemotherapy schedule agreed and the treatment plan moving forward and everything clear in his and his wife's minds, Dan now wanted to tell his boys about his illness and forthcoming treatments.

Lewis, being the eldest, of an age and having the level of intelligence to understand, got full chapter and verse. His first question to his dad was "When does it start?" Dan explained the dates and timescales, explaining furthermore his need to get all the information together before telling his son. Dan also made his eldest offspring promise that if he had ANY questions, to ask him or his mum and not to Google anything. Google can be the enemy in some situations, and this definitely was considered one of them. Lewis agreed.

Telling Ollie, the youngest, was going to be a very different conversation.

Dan explained carefully that he needed some medicine to get rid of some bad cells, and if he had any worries about anything to ask his parents.

"Now, this medicine might make me tired and feel poorly and make my hair fall out." Ollie's response was classic: "Well, that's just stupid – having a medicine that makes you poorly. Can I go on the Xbox now?"

Dan had to smile, there was one happy and so far completely unfazed fella.

Dan felt happier knowing his boys now knew about his illness and what the immediate future might hold. It meant that things could be talked about – perhaps not completely openly, but he didn't have to try to hide what was going on. They were a family, Team Cook, and they were in this together.

The best news to both boys was that yes, the family was still going on holiday to Cornwall the following week. A place where Dan and his family knew they could completely relax and disconnect for a while.

Might Make You Smile
BOWEL CLASS NOT BOWLS CLASS

With so many side effects from two different types of cancer so far, Julie was used to some re-education; and learning to live with her body. It was only when she found that her bowels – which had been an issue even prior to her cancer diagnosis – started to be affected by her medication, that she was recommended a 'Bowel Re-education Class'. At first, she thought her Macmillan nurse was joking with her, but it was true; there was help and assistance for anyone who was experiencing difficulties in the toilet department.

A week after talking to her nurse, and after spending a particularly miserable weekend at home unable to venture out as the pain and discomfort of not being able to go to the toilet at all, and by Monday was feeling like she was going to explode, she contacted her treatment centre. She found out when the next bowel therapy session was scheduled, she had just a couple of days to wait. By the time the morning of the session came, Julie was more than ready. Her discomfort was almost unbearable and she knew if she didn't do anything, it was likely she would have to be admitted to hospital for manual assistance. A non-too-pleasant experience and one she was definitely keen to avoid.

Julie arrived for the session and was comforted to see she was not alone, in fact there was quite a full class already in the waiting room. Julie took a seat, and she almost burst out laughing as another person taking the session was the double of the late Barbara Woodhouse, dog trainer extraordinaire. Neat haircut, sensible shoes, a tweed skirt, with a no-nonsense expression fixed firmly on her face. Julie had watched many a programme featuring the canine genius bringing unruly four-legged furry friends in line, and then rewarding them only when they had mastered her commands.

The attendees filed into the large, airy room, which was filled with multi-coloured yoga mats, all spaced equally apart. In one firmly spoken command, each mat was claimed by a delegate. Julie listened to the instructions for relaxation exercises, visualisation, and techniques of how to approach the tricky business of going to the toilet. At first, the embarrassment was palpable, but as the session progressed everyone seemed to relax, and what Julie was hearing made sense. She had never considered 'pushing only from the hips', but it made perfect sense now. The relaxation techniques were already beginning to work, when the mechanics of the body were explained, and how everything from food, mood, anxiety, as well as medication, can affect the simplest of bodily functions; it was hardly surprising that she was having difficulties and things become stalled. A body, she was informed, cannot be trained to do things on command; unlike a dog thought Julie.

Julie rid herself of the image of the therapist standing in front of her enunciating in a clear voice 'Sit' accompanied by the legendary Barbara Woodhouse arm gesture, which every dog obeyed regardless. She stifled a laugh at the image of all the attendees sitting obediently. By the end of the session, Julie felt relaxed and more in control than ever. Getting home, and in the comfort of her own bathroom, Julie was granted the release she had been longing for. She vowed never again to mock the benefits of her 'Bowel Class', in fact, she would go on a 'Bowel Class' promotional tour, starting with her next support group meeting, she was a convert.

Good For A Grin
ROID RAGE

It was only when Roger had allowed himself ten minutes to read the warning leaflet that came with his steroids did he find it a real page turner.

By all accounts he could have all or any of almost fifty different side effects. The steroid was given to help his body repair itself, particularly after chemotherapy. He had been taking it for almost five weeks now. When he thought of it like that he realised he had, so far, been lucky, having had none of the nasty side effects. Yes, it was fair to say Roger was feeling a little smug with his findings.

The Commonwealth Games was on the television and as he wasn't working he decided he would spend the afternoon watching the day's events. Just as he was settling down into his comfortable chair, his wife brought him a cup of tea.

"Thought I'd watch some of the Games," he said, taking the cup from her.

"There's the netball finals on next," she smiled.

Deciding he had nothing to lose, Roger got comfy. It was England versus Australia. Now Roger wasn't a true follower of the sport, it had to be said, and yet he couldn't help but get caught up in the fast-paced, dramatic match. He had been warned that the steroids prescribed to aid his recovery could make him a little moody, irritable even, and possibly a little bombastic on occasion.

His wife, however, had been completely honest with him and told him she had seen absolutely no change. Until that is, the netball match. By the middle of it Roger was almost standing on his chair screaming for England to win. Both teams were playing out of their skins. The countdown clock was ticking, and Roger was by now jumping up and down, the air blue. His wife was a little shocked, she had no idea Roger even knew those words, so she steered well clear of the lounge. With the last second to go, England scored a final point. The game ended 52 – 51, England won Gold.

By this time Roger was hoarse. His wife stood in the doorway, wearing a look of both shock and relief – the game had ended.

Roger climbed down from his standing position on the armchair, smiled as he walked past his wife. "Time for a beer I think," he called as he passed her.

"Mmmm… think perhaps those steroids may be taking effect after all," she called after him. She quickly turned off the television and followed her husband into the kitchen. The victory for England was history-making, 2018 would definitely be a year to remember. Roger's wife thought about this as she straightened the furniture. As she passed through the room, she admitted to herself that she was just pleased that only the chair, nor anything else, had been broken.

Might Make You Smile
THE SWIMMING HAT BRIGADE

Helen had succumbed to her treatment. She had good days, and she had bad days. One thing was constant however, her support network. Her girls, Helen's Heroes, were always there for her. Some days she felt like she needed to be surrounded by their constant babble, raucous laughter, and often insane anecdotes; and others she preferred no company or the company of just one. Helen's Heroes was made up of the women she had met through playgroups, having children, living in the same neighbourhood, work, life in general and some being single mums like her; all having shared life's experiences with her at various points. Dealing with cancer was no exception. As soon as Helen had broken the news, the Heroes rallied around.

Helen made the decision to have her hair cut short, having sported long tresses for quite some time. She had also decided to try the 'cold cap' method while having chemotherapy in the hope of avoiding hair loss. This entailed a gel-filled cap being worn before, during, and after chemotherapy. It was by no means the most glamorous of looks, but one Helen was going to give a go. A girl's night in was planned at Helen's house, and a theme was decided, unbeknown to her. With drinks and nibbles organised, Helen waited for the arrival of her dearest friends.

The doorbell rang, and Helen completed one last check of her appearance in the mirror. She was slowly beginning to get used to her shorn appearance and her hair was surviving for the moment. The lamplight around the front door was reflecting something as she opened it and for a moment she was blinded. It was then she saw each of her friends; as they stepped over the threshold they all sported shiny, hairless heads. Helen couldn't help but laugh at the multi-coloured heads. Everyone was sporting a swimming cap of one description or another; faces pulled tight at obscure angles, and none looking like themselves. It was safe to say that Helen sported the longest hairstyle that evening, and the group laughed long and hard into the early hours at each other's bizarre appearance. The photos of their escapades were circulated and enjoyed for weeks to come. Helen couldn't help but laugh to herself whenever she remembered her group of friends and how they made her laugh so much that night.

Good For A Grin
ENTER RONNIE

Pat had begun his treatment. His surgery, to give him what was commonly referred to as 'Barbie Bum', courtesy of being diagnosed with rectal cancer, had been completed.

His rehabilitation with the help of his wife, best friend and soulmate Paula was ticking along nicely. There were of course the odd bumps in the recovery road, but Paula and Pat navigated their way around them as best they could. They were both making adjustments to carry on as best they could with normal life, but were determined not to allow their lives to be defined by cancer, the treatments or any other aspect of their current situation. They were both of the opinion that 'life is life' , and not matter what it threw at you, the alternative of no life at all was far worse.

Pat and Paula had always loved eating out; they had favourite restaurants, and hotels they loved to stay at, but also loved exploring and trying out new places and cuisines.

Having had the surgery on what was already a painful bum – a true 'pain in the arse' (pun absolutely intended) – Pat had purchased a comfort ring, the sort of device used by anyone from pregnant women to haemorrhoid sufferers. It was a state-of-the-art, memory foam jobbie that had been recommended for his recovery from surgery.. A real Rolls-Royce of derriere indulgence.

At first Pat had said he would never be taking 'Ronnie' – the name given to the ring by Paula, now held with a modicum of affection after they had grown close – out in public, but as time went on and he and Paula settled into their new life, it seemed less and less of an issue. A date was chosen, they were going to enjoy a lunch out. Ronnie was coming too.

Pat, even prior to his diagnosis, had been very much a 'get on with it' kind of guy. This attitude didn't change when he was told he had cancer. There was a quote from Charles R. Swindoll that he liked to live by: "Life is ten percent what happens to you and ninety percent how you react to it."

Ronnie had a bag of his own, which looked like any other you might take shopping. The restaurant Pat and Paula chose was perfect and their lunch date long awaited. Thinking ahead, they had already discussed how they would co-ordinate the delicate ring manoeuvre so as not to draw attention. Being keen ballroom and Latin dancers, they possessed the skills to easily execute this minor 'quick step'.

As they were shown to their table they were delighted with their choice – so far, so good. When Paula took her seat discreetly she slipped the bag under the table, and, in one effortlessly fluid movement the ring was on Pat's chair and he was sitting comfortably. In fact, he delighted in feeling a little smug when he realised that without the ring his seating position would not have been great for him anyway. And so a lovely lunch was enjoyed, Ronnie unseen yet offering the greatest of comfort. Strictly Come Dancing had nothing on these two.

Might Make You Smile
H.H.C.
(HAPPY HERCEPTIN CATTLE)

Anita was still trying to come to terms with the new person she had become. It was an undeniable fact that cancer had changed her. Although some would say this was inevitable, it was so much easier to brush the emotional as well as the physical change off as being 'one of those things', unless you are the person actually living it. Treatment days were often anxious times accompanied by their own levels of stress. She had been prescribed the drug Herceptin, and had to attend hospital to have it administered. It was delivered by special courier and was administered immediately.

On this particular day Anita was feeling a little low, but as she walked into the treatment room her spirits lifted slightly. Everyone, from the nursing staff to the patients, had the ability to bring the room alive with positivity. They were all there for the same goal; Herceptin was going to help make them better. Looking around Anita couldn't help but smile to herself. All of the patients were either hooked up to saline drips, which helped to keep them hydrated and keep vital veins open for the life giving treatment, or in the process of being fitted with I.Vs in readiness for the much anticipated delivery.

Information drifted through that the delivery was going to be a little late, which had the knock-on effect of numerous loo breaks. The room took on a cattle market atmosphere as overloaded bladders, skipping rope length I.V. systems with accompanying wheeled monitors, and nurses attempting to assist with the great contortionist acts that are patients attempting to go to the toilet after waiting in line attached to their I.V.s. There was an almost synchronised dance of patients and nurses keeping the I.V.lines intact, and the assistance of releasing clothing in cubicles that felt no bigger than telephone boxes. It would only take one of the 'cattle' to get the giggles, and there was the distinct possibility of disaster.

Times like these reminded Anita of the camaraderie that is experienced by even the most subdued person. She found her spirits lifted by the end of the treatment sessions, and it was ironic that the benefits of her treatment were not just drug-related. Herceptin was her elixir of life, but the connections and friendships made while sitting amongst others enduring the same treatment and their collective fight with cancer, she knew would last her a lifetime, and she couldn't help but feel grateful.

Good For A Grin
SAVING THOSE SWIMMERS

Dan and Nat had NO plans to have any more children, their adored two sons Lewis and Ollie being more than capable of keeping them constantly on their toes. It had been recommended to Dan that saving some sperm was a sensible idea, as chemotherapy had the nasty habit of making people sterile. There could, in the future, be the question "Why didn't you do it?" if he had chosen not to take the advice.

Once agreed, Dan was referred to the andrology department at Hammersmith Hospital. Having never made a sperm deposit before, this was a tad nerve-racking and most definitely uncharted territory. After dropping youngest son Ollie off at school, Dan and Nat made their way to the hospital. Dan did wonder whether her accompanying him was more for the amusement factor than perhaps a purely supportive role – the look of sheer horror on the face of every bloke in the waiting room when they sat down was a sight. Was that a smile he saw pass over her lips?

Having filled out a ton of paperwork, Dan was present with 'the cup'. The extremely efficient-looking nurse announced "Room one, Mr. Cook," closely followed by, "There are magazines in the drawer, or a DVD if you wish." This information was delivered in the same manner as an assistant at Tesco might direct you to the flour in the baking section. Avoiding eye contact with anyone, Dan made his way to the room.

He had absolutely no intentions of touching anything in that room. It was one of those situations where this was definitely one of the last places he wanted to be, but he knew it needed to be done.

Magazine? No thank you, he wasn't going anywhere near that drawer, let alone its contents. He dreaded to think who had been at either.

DVD? That would mean touching a remote control. Ugh! No, that wasn't happening either.

Good old imagination was the order of the day – it never fails. Deposit made, job done. Dan's mind screamed, "Get me out of here," closely followed by his body and his wife. That was part one of the job done anyway. Yes, to add a little insult to injury they like you to repeat the procedure. Two deposits, please.

That is for another day.

Might Make You Smile
LUCKY BLACK CATS?

There it was again. The small black cat popped its head around the bottom of Jan's bed and regarded her quizzically with its jade eyes. Jan watched as the cat slowly wound its tail around the leg of the bed. All of this may not have been quite so noteworthy if it wasn't for the fact that Jan's current place of residence was the tenth floor of Addenbrooke's Hospital, lovingly referred to the 'Penthouse Suite'.

The cat turned again to look at her for a moment before she saw another small black furry head, and then another. In the space of a couple of minutes Jan had counted five more cats. She burst out laughing when she watched two cats face each other and raise a paw in what appeared to be a feline 'high five', and then proceed to walk up the wall opposite Jan's bed. They were almost to the ceiling and standing perfectly horizontal to the floor, as if it were a normal, everyday occurrence.

Next, two more cats, which had been sitting around the leg of the bed watching with equal fascination as Jan had, at the other wall walking cats, then followed the first pair. Jan could not believe her eyes and turned to talk to the patient in the bed next to her but she was fast asleep, snoring gently, oblivious to the amazing spectacle. Jan returned to watch the final pair follow the other four. By now the first four were upside down on the ceiling, looking like the most unlikely of light fittings.

Halfway up the wall, the final pair of cats turned and faced Jan, and she could have sworn they waved at her with a single paw each before continuing on their way up to join the others. When all of the cats were together again as a group, they sat down in an upside down circle, their tails dangling in midair, resembling furry question marks. By now Jan was laughing so much she was almost crying.

Nurse Cath could see Jan laughing heartily, she felt happy that even though Jan had recently received a bone marrow transplant, she hadn't lost her sense of humour and was clearly finding something amusing. Nurse Cath made her way to Jan's bed, and smiled at her carer. "Have you ever seen anything like this?" She asked pointing to the ceiling, the cats watching Jan and Nurse Cath with heads to one side. Nurse Cath smiled at her patient, she had worked in Addenbrooke's Oncology department for years now and had listened to many stories of fantastical goings on, particularly during certain treatments, but black cats scaling the walls? Six black cats scaling the walls at that! Yes, that was a new one on her. Hallucinations came in all shapes and sizes, but this was a first.

Good For A Grin
OLYMPIC HOPES

Mike had managed to keep his diagnosis quiet from his work colleagues for some time. He felt well enough to work and had somehow managed to navigate his life around appointments, treatments and symptoms. As his appearance wasn't affected too much, cancer often being a 'silent' illness, he carried on with life as normally as possible, feeling this was the approach that worked best for him in dealing with his cancer.

It was only when he started taking steroids as part of his treatment that his appearance changed dramatically. When his face began to swell, and he got the full measure of the 'moon face' side effects, he knew he could not keep his illness to himself any longer. Being a sales executive for an office furniture company, and constantly meeting clients and suppliers face-to-face, he was slightly concerned for his work.

In fact he had no cause to be worried, and when the news was revealed there was nothing but full support from everyone, from the managing director down.

The head office for his employer was very near the Russian Embassy in London. There was a conference to be attended by all sales staff, and Mike was looking forward to getting together and catching up with everyone he didn't often get to see in person. It was a great team-building event too, and forged relationships no end.

He knew there would be questions asked, but he was prepared and looking forward to the 'after conference' fun of socialising with some great friends and colleagues.

The conference was a busy affair, with lots of speakers, target projections and new product lines showcased. Mike sat with the other regional sales executives and happily joked about the steroid treatment and how he could outperform any athlete in strength and speed, laughing that at that moment in time he would fail a drug test spectacularly.

At lunch time a large group of the sales staff ventured out to take in a little of what central London had to offer. As the group passed the Russian Embassy, one of Mike's colleagues shouted across the group, "Mike, quick, get yourself in there; you'll be signed up in a heartbeat for the next Olympics. You'll be a sensation, no questions asked." The group fell about laughing. Mike agreed, "Ah, yes, my Olympic dreams would come true after all."

The group proceeded to take bets on Mike's chances in each organised event. It was agreed that with his steroid intake he could beat all comers, including the entire Russian team. Mike was an athletic superstar without even stepping foot on a track. An enthusiastic and highly amusing lunch was taken by the group.

Might Make You Smile
CHICK CHICK HAIR

Clare's six-year-old daughter had been her tonic throughout her cancer journey. Although she had initially struggled with Clare's hair loss – much more so than Clare herself or even her beauty conscious, hairdressing family – she gradually came around to the dramatic change in her mother's appearance.

For the first couple of months, after Clare had finally lost all of her hair, her daughter would insist Clare wear a hat at all times, even indoors. Although on occasion this could prove a little uncomfortable – it was amazing how hot a head could get indoors covered with a hat – Clare was more than happy to oblige anything while her daughter came to terms with things in her mind.

Eventually, the little girl became more and more at ease with her mother's bald head. When the first regrowth came through, her daughter would pat the warm fuzz calling it 'baby chick, chick hair'.

For Clare, it was a huge comfort that her daughter was adapting to the changes in her life, and doing so with the humour and outlook that only a six-year-old could.

Good For A Grin
PUMPS, RINGS AND ALL MANNER OF THINGS

Sam never thought he would ever be thinking about erectile dysfunction, let alone experiencing it. Initially he was almost in denial. This wasn't like a 'blip' caused by over indulgence on the beer front or not being 'in the mood'. This was dysfunction on another level, a completely flacid fella. What man wants to acknowledge that, ever?

It was only when he met other men in the same position at a support session at Maggie's (cancer support centre) that he allowed himself to acknowledge the problem. It is said that recognising there is a problem is half the way to solving it. Well, this sentiment was perhaps slightly ambitious, but he felt he was certainly ready to deal with the matter.

There was a lot of humour in the group. It was then that Sam began to realise that this was so often the case when men got together – they make fun of a serious subject, and end up even poking fun at themselves. This was how men dealt with so many problems. Once all the barriers were down it was so much easier. Before long, talk of lubricants, rings to help with maintaining an erection and a whole bunch of other aids that could be tried was free flowing. Sam laughed with the rest of the group.

The huge weight he had been carrying around after his run-in with cancer had been lifted. Armed with newly acquired information, some aids, even a few top tips you were not going to find in any medical leaflet, he felt happier than he had in what seemed like an age. Sex was for having fun, it had just lost the fun part when there was a bump in the road. Sam knew he had to approach getting things back on track with fun too, learn to find the playful part of 'getting back in the saddle'. He was sure the rest would follow.

Sam knew his partner had already shown she was happy to wait, be patient and that he needed to come to terms with things in his own way. Well, he was in a good place now and there was a sense to make the effort on his part.

He passed a florists and bought a dozen red roses, then a bottle of champagne. And with his bag of 'goodies' and information that he had acquired, he was going to put phase one of his newly formed plan into action. The main aim was to remind the love of his life that this was still very much what she was. The rest would take time and patience, but it would all be dealt with as something to enjoy, and he was sure together they would do just that.

Instead of feeling like he was in some way failing, he now felt like he was almost being naughty, even laughing to himself at what he had planned. He marvelled at how a situation, if thought of in a completely different manner, can suddenly work for you. His 'bag of tricks' felt more like 'toys' now, and that in itself made him feel all the more 'up for it'.

Sam had learnt of other methods like pumps that could be fitted if his 'toys' didn't work, but for now he was happy to take the first baby steps and have fun trying them out. Having fun trying things out together was the important first step.

Might Make You Smile
NEW HAIRDO GRANDMA?

Polly was spending time with her family, she was staying the weekend with her son and his family. One morning she was getting herself dressed, trying to make herself look presentable, when her grandson toddled in. Chemotherapy had left Polly with hair regrowth that was finally beginning to make an appearance, but until her hair was completely regrown she had decided on a wig which helped her feel a little more comfortable.

As her grandson stood in the doorway, Polly waited for his reaction to seeing her not wearing her wig; it was hanging neatly on the bedpost. This was the first time he had seen her without it and she felt a small rise of anxiety waiting for him to say something. She wondered if her appearance frightened him or made him uneasy, because she had no intention of upsetting her beloved grandchild.

Smiling broadly at his grandma, the little boy tipped his head to one side looking quizzical and then ran toward Polly, his arms outstretched. "New haircut, Grandma?" he asked pointing at the downy regrowth. Polly laughed and scooped the little boy up in her arms. Then he reached for the wig, promptly popped it on his own head, and ran back to the mirror where Polly was sitting. Turning this way and that they laughed at his reflection.

After a few moments, he turned to Polly and declared that although he liked his Grandma's new haircut, he loved the shiny wig. After that morning together Polly's grandson would often ask her if she was feeling well, his concern evident for her. She found his demeanour both touching and charming. As her treatment went on, it was her young grandson who always had the ability to make her smile.

Good For A Grin
TAKE A SEAT
(WOULD IF I COULD)

When every part of your body, after being provided with a 'barbie bum', and everybody around you (including your consultant), says you can't sit still for too long, you have to listen.

There remains, however, the fact that you have to attend appointments. Being unable to drive is one thing, but not being able to actually sit in a car is a major hurdle too.

Pat found himself in this predicament. He needed to attend various appointments but knew he was in no fit state to sit through the journey. Rectal surgery will do that to you. It remains a pain in the arse for quite some time (excuse the pun).

Paula was more than happy to drive her husband wherever he needed to be, but it still didn't solve the actual problem of how he was going to get to those places, literally.

Pat then came up with an idea: he would have to lie across the back seat of Paula's car.. Then when they arrived at their destination he would have to effectively 'back out' of the car. It would be an understatement to say Pat and Paula laughed out loud at what they must have looked like on the various CCTVs that hospitals and medical centres delighted in having in vast numbers in their grounds and car parks.

They could imagine the scene:

So, woman pulls up in car. Checks her mirrors, taking note of who is around, the fewer spectators the better. The coast is clear. Trying not to look furtive she then gets out and opens the rear driver's-side door. Very slowly, ever so carefully, a man extricates himself from the back seat, feet, legs and bottom first until he is standing.

Pat and Paula often wondered what those monitoring the cameras must have thought of the sight.

Was this a form of punishment for the husband? Perhaps a little something they liked to do for kicks? Had the husband lost a bet and this was the forfeit or, heaven forbid, had he left the toilet seat up one too many times? Alternatively, had she kidnapped him? Although, kidnapping someone per se was not entirely improbable, but then taking them to a local hospital…? Not so much.

The list went on and on and provided countless amusing moments.

Might Make You Smile
IS THAT YOU DAD? OR IS THAT ME?

Clare loved looking back at family photos. Although her appearance had changed dramatically, particularly since the diagnosis of cancer, she wasn't in any way bothered by her altered appearance. She had lost her hair to chemotherapy but had found the process character building. She knew and felt she was more, so much more, than the sum of her hair. As lovely as hair was, she was more proud of her attitude towards herself. She did have a wig which she loved but rarely wore, preferring to be free of any encumbrance. She was even happy to attend family outings and gatherings, not minding if photos were taken.

As it turned out, on occasion, this sometimes caused some confusion; especially when recollecting and reminiscing over family photos. This point was highlighted when her practically bald, seventy-something year old father quizzically looked at one particular snap and questioned why he was at that particular gathering. He couldn't understand why he had no recollection of the day at all, or why he would have even been there. Clare pointed out that the bald person in the picture was in fact herself, and teased him as to how he couldn't recognise his own daughter, feigning shock and disappointment.

She was in fact delighted, finding the whole situation highly amusing. It had often been commented on by family and friends just how much Clare resembled her father, clearly she had never realised how true this was.

Good For A Grin
"CASHIER NUMBER TWO PLEASE." ACTUALLY, DEPOSIT NUMBER TWO

With the holiday date looming ever closer, Dan was aware he had a limited timetable to get his second sperm deposit done at Hammersmith.

He was up first thing and at the andrology department when it opened. Hardly a January sale type of affair, but he needed to be one of the first in. More paperwork, several blokes sitting around looking decidedly uncomfortable, zero eye contact. This was definitely not a meet-up at the local boozer kind of place, no light-hearted banter or discussing the football or rugby scores. Nat didn't accompany him on this occasion; Dan mused that the other occupants had no idea what they were spared.

Room number two this time. Maybe these places could do with the same announcer as used in banks and post offices: "Cashier number two, please". Same drill as before. Dan avoided the drawer with the 'magazines' and the option of the DVD. Imagination ruled, job done, once again Dan signed the paperwork and was out the door in record time.

He was told he would have to go back at some point for a consultation, but until that consultation happened nobody was allowed to use the sperm, including Dan!

That consultation could wait for another day, Dan decided, as he headed off for further tests to clear the way for the much anticipated family holiday, where talk of treatments, side effects and everything other than enjoying family life, creating memories and great times could be forgotten.

Might Make You Smile
RUNNING AWAY WITH YOU

Sadie had tried everything to keep from losing her hair during her cancer treatment, but to no avail. She had resigned herself to the inevitable and purchased a fabulous wig which made her feel a little better about the loss of her much loved tresses. When she spoke to her husband Al about the loss and what he thought she would look like having short or even no hair, he simply replied that Sadie had a pretty face and would resemble either an older Sinead O'Connor, or a young Judith Chalmers. A compliment indeed.

Sadie wasn't a person to dwell on the negatives in life. She was happy to chat and joke about the variety of indignities one went through when dealing with cancer, and she often regaled her listeners with her daily musings. The hair loss meant she became completely hair free. Which she joked with her listeners resulted in no more waxing, shaving, or plucking; and as her energy levels had somewhat depleted that was fine by her. She hoped if she shared her thoughts and feelings with her BBC Essex Radio listeners, she would show and encourage others that there can still be life with cancer.

It was a cooler day at the beginning of Autumn, and Sadie had finished her radio show, and knew she needed to pop into her local Tesco to grab something for dinner that evening. She found she was a little more prone to forgetfulness since her treatments, and removing something from the freezer for meals was, more often than not, something she forgot.

As Sadie stepped over the supermarket threshold, she was greeted by the warm blast of air from within the supermarket. Sadie had an idea what she wanted and quickly headed to the aisles picking up a favourite main course and dessert. As she turned towards the checkout, Sadie was aware that her hands were wet, not just a little damp, but truly wet. After a second she felt what had caused the spectacle, her nose was running like a tap turned on full; not just a momentary drip, it was in full gush. Sadie had nothing to stop her nose, not tissue, nothing; not even her sleeve could stem the flow. Wearing a leather jacket meant she had nothing more than a very damp 'snail trail' as she tried desperately to shield her embarrassment.

By now she was at the checkout, thankfully there was no queue. 'I'm so sorry,' apologised Sadie, from behind her sleeve. 'I don't even have a tissue,' she laughed. The checkout lady grinned at Sadie, she knew who she was, and often listened to her radio show before starting her shift at the supermarket. She reached under the counter and located a packet of tissues. She popped them on top of Sadie's shopping, and then scooped all of the shopping into a carrier bag for the presenter. Smiling, she hooked the shopping bag onto Sadie's free hand, 'love your show'. She smiled as Sadie left the shop, her arm still across her face looking for all the world like a pantomime villain, all she needed was a black cape, only her eyes visible over her arm.

As soon as Sadie was free of the cosy interior, she felt the dripping ease and quickly located the tissues. Not having to shave your legs was great, but who knew there was a purpose for nasal hair. Sadie was roaring with laughter, barely coherent, as she regaled Al with the tale over dinner. She looked forward to sharing it again with her listeners the following morning.

Good For A Grin
DIFFUSE LARGE B CELL NON-HODGKIN'S LYMPHOMA

That title is quite a mouthful, as was the number of pills Peter was now taking to combat his run-in with this type of cancer.

Being a man with what could be considered a slightly warped sense of humour, he took the new additions to his daily routine in his stride. The treatment plan he was placed on meant he had two doses of chemotherapy via I.V., the 'Gin and Tonic' sessions, as he liked to call them, followed by a smorgasbord of multi-coloured pills taken on a daily basis – these, he was convinced, made him sound like a rattlesnake, and he joked that he was afraid to fart in case he blew the seat off his jeans and peppered the cats with psychedelic NHS buckshot.

Along with a good dose of prednisolone for added umph, he felt there was a very real danger of casualties of both animal and human variety should he get close and let one rip.

Living on the edge of farmland, Peter thought a walk in the back garden, keeping an eye out for local wildlife of course, was perhaps the safest option. He checked first for any neighbours who might have had similar intentions – going out into the garden, that is, not preparing to break wind.

He had no intention of appearing on the news under the headline: "Local man arrested for causing assault with deadly fart."

What Peter wasn't expecting was that the chemo via I.V. would make him feel pretty trippy, and it has to be said he did comment that he felt a little 'on cloud nine' at times. His wife likened his behaviour to having a nine-year-old hyperactive boy in the house again. Amusing for an hour or two; utter exhaustion setting in after any longer.

As with any 'up' there must be a 'down'. This followed a day or two later when the nine-year-old boy became the sullen 'emo' teenager.

Peter and his wife being in their retirement years made for an interesting time, certainly never dull. Yes, Peter, Sue, their cats and dogs had to learn to adjust to their new life, but this they did with a certain degree of laughter and humour.

Might Make You Smile
OOOH! I LOVE YOUR HAIRDO

For some reason, Jenny was a little embarrassed wearing her wig. She had undergone hours of debilitating treatment. Chemotherapy had robbed her of her hair, her eyebrows, and even leg hair, for which she was delighted; no more shaving.

For whatever reason though, she couldn't resign herself to wearing a wig. She felt she almost had to explain its presence, in an apologetic manner; as if to say 'sorry, you don't mind if my wig accompanies me today, do you?'

Jenny decided, if she wore it as often as possible she would begin to feel more comfortable about it. With this in mind, she wore the wig every time she stepped out of the house. This definitely seemed to help her feel more comfortable, but it was one particular trip to the supermarket that made her feel truly at peace with her hairpiece.

On a mundane trip with her daughter, while the food was being packed away at the checkout, Jenny noticed the cashier was an old friend, someone she had not seen for quite some time, but who had been part of a bigger circle of friends previous to her diagnosis and treatment.

'Hi Cath, how are you?', smiled Jenny. The woman looked up, and recognition spread across her face. 'Why Jenny, how are you? Gosh, it's been years since I saw you last.'

'I know! I'm good, thank you.' Jenny didn't feel the need to divulge her recent woes, she was happy to just indulge the need to chat.

'You look fabulous. Now that I know it's you I have to ask, where did you get your hair cut?' Cath was passing items through the scanner as she waited for Jenny to reply. Jenny paused for a moment before replying, 'It's a wig.'

'That's fantastic! What a great idea, wigs are all the rage at the moment. You can change your look without constant trips to the hairdresser.' Cath enthused.

Again, Jenny didn't feel the need to explain further. It was Cath that broke the pause in conversation. 'Can you give me the name of where you got it?' Cath then went on to briefly explain that she had just finished treatment for breast cancer, and although she enjoyed wearing a headscarf – something Jenny hadn't even noticed – she had now found the hairstyle she liked, Jenny's, and would love a wig just like it.

On the drive back home, Jenny realised upon reflection that she had become consumed with her own insecurities. She was not always completely aware of those around her, and by wearing her wig, she had actually proven inspirational to a friend who, as it turned out, had been on a similar cancer journey herself.

Jenny also began to realise that, if she looked at her wig as a fashion accessory no different to a bag, scarf, or jewellery, she could maybe even have some fun with it. Maybe, she mused, she would try a red shoulder length bob next, or even a brunette. The possibilities were endless.

Good For A Grin
NOT EXACTLY NICKY CLARKE

Myer had been an oncology nurse for ten years. During this time she had been involved with and nursed people through all aspects of cancer and oncology treatments.

There was only one thing, one simple aspect, which she dreaded more than anything: helping people shave their heads. Although she dreaded it, she never refused, and sometimes it was even where the most fun was to be had.

One particular occasion, when she was called upon for her most feared task, was with a young man of about twenty who had suffered hair loss as soon as he started his chemotherapy treatment. He was studying to be a dentist, 6' 2" and weighed 100 kilos – not a small man by any means.

This young man's hair was a mass of thick curls and he needed it all gone. But before it was removed he wanted to have some fun. Myer, as always, was a tad nervous. The young man asked if she could shave it first of all into a Mohawk style. Myer promised she would do her best but couldn't guarantee the results. The patient took pictures on his mobile phone throughout the process, with he and Myer laughing at all the weird stages his hair went through as it was being removed.

Myer was the first to admit she was no Nicky Clarke, but between them and the fits of laughter, the result was pretty impressive.

The young man sent pictures to his mates, and then in a flash he sent one last picture to his mother. With that done, the none-too-small and somewhat imposing man quickly asked for the Mohawk to be shaved off completely, before his mum arrived and truly told him off. His friends were very impressed with his somewhat short-lived hairstyle. His mother…not so much.

Might Make You Smile
DROP DEAD GORGEOUS

Michelle had been through countless chemotherapy treatments, and some of the treatments had been carried out at home. The nurses came to the house; often they were ladies, and the treatments would take anything from three to four hours.

Michelle was sitting at home, waiting patiently for her nurse to arrive when there was a knock at the door. Michelle opened the door to a 'wonderful surprise'; there stood a very handsome young man. He had a leather jacket slung over his shoulder, and he was wearing Aviator sunglasses, looking for all the world like Tom Cruise in 'Top Gun'. The accompanying soundtrack was already in Michelle's mind as the song 'Take My Breath Away' broke into her thoughts. The young man cheerily asked for Michelle. Michelle replied eagerly 'That's me.' Sounding a little too enthusiastic for what was not a particularly pleasant procedure. 'My name's Rob, and I'm your chemo nurse.' He said, smiling.

With that, Michelle grabbed him and pulled him inside. He was so attentive, and drop dead gorgeous, that Michelle couldn't help herself; secretly texting her two single sisters, complete with surreptitious picture and a brief description of his attributes.

One of Michelle's sisters lived a good thirty minute drive away in another town, and the other one worked flexible hours and was at home, again a distance away. Within twenty five minutes of the text being sent, two cars could be heard screeching around the corner and coming to a skidding halt outside. Michelle watched as her sisters near sprinted up the garden path, in a race to get to the house first. Almost falling through the front door, the pair bundled into the house. One rushed to the bathroom, where Michelle could hear hairspray, deodorant, and perfume being liberally applied. The other wasted no time, and seized the opportunity to immediately ply the poor man with copious amounts of tea, coffee, biscuits, and anything else she could come up with.

Sister number one suddenly burst from the bathroom, looking like she was going on a night out, primped and preened to within an inch of her life, and surrounded by a cloud of hair product and perfume.

Michelle marvelled at the poor fella, he was so polite, and blushing. As he finished what he had come to do, he sat down on the sofa, a rookie mistake. In a flash, the two sisters had squeezed either side of him, and began firing countless questions as to his dating eligibility.

He took it all in good humour, and was very accommodating; Michelle guessed this wasn't the first time he had attracted such attention. What was normally a somewhat miserable day took on a distinctive cheerier note, and everyone left smiling.

Good For A Grin
BACK TO BLACK

When Dan realised his hair was falling out he knew he had to take measures. Going along to his barbers he explained his predicament.

In no time the clippers were out and expertly wielded – that was it, Dan was hair-free! It certainly didn't look like him staring back in the mirror. He knew instantly he would never really like it, him being bald just didn't sit right in his mind, but it did make the whole anxiety of hair loss a bit less intimidating. There were, after all, countless men sporting buzzcuts by choice.

Dan also knew that after his treatment and his hair had grown back he would not be one of those. Although many people commented on how much the hair-free look suited him, it wasn't him. Mind you, the barber not charging for the cut was a nice way of softening the blow.

Dan's mates, in true mate fashion, more than made up for that by continuing to take the piss, along with taking bets as to whether his hair would grow back curly, straight, or even… ginger! Suffice to say they were disappointed when in fact it did not. Though it did grow back in his normal shade (but with a little more grey than he remembered, that absolutely must have been a chemo effect…), it was so baby soft, so touchably, run your fingers through it soft, that he was convinced he could have done a Johnson's Baby Shampoo advert… nice!

Might Make You Smile
TREATMENT TAG TEAM

Lesley was all set. Mel, her best friend, was pregnant in Dubai and was unable to fly home to Cambridgeshire when the news came through that both her parents had to undergo cancer treatments. Lynne was due to come home after her double mastectomy the same day Don had to be in hospital for a treatment for his own cancer. Lesley was Mel's closest friend, and her parents were like family, so there was no question as to who could help out at such a distressing time.

Mel's mum, Lynne, had been diagnosed with breast cancer, while Mel's dad, Don, was being treated for bowel cancer. What were the odds, that on the same date Lynne was due to be allowed home after her surgery Don would be undergoing a procedure himself?

The day arrived when Lesley was due to take care of both Lynne and Don; she had everything organised with military precision. With Mel in Dubai, Lesley had been keeping her constantly updated with her parents progress. Don had driven himself to Addenbrooke's for his treatment, assuring her he was more than capable of the drive.

Lesley had arrived at the huge hospital, and had quickly located both wards; as luck would have it they were at opposite ends of the vast hospital. Lesley was armed with gifts of chocolate for both her charges, a fine continental selection for Lynn and a multi-packet of Walnut Whips for Don, being at a loss as to what to buy him, and still questioning her dubious choice as she made her way through the corridors of the hospital.

Lesley had known Mel and her parents for years, and she was apprehensive as to how both would be after their respective procedures.

The hospital was hot, and she was already beginning to feel a little sweaty and flustered. She made her way to the ward where she knew Lynne had a room. The nurse showed her where Lynne's room was, and Lesley mentally prepared herself before entering. Popping her head around the door, she was greeted by the smiling, beautifully presented and impeccably made-up Lynne, looking as fabulous as ever, if a little stiff in her movements due to her dressings. Lesley was openly amused, and relief flooded through her. Lynne beamed at her, and gently patted the space beside her on the bed for Lesley to sit down.

"Darling, thank you so much for coming, this really is too much, you having to take care of us both like this." Lynne explained she was waiting to see the consultant, and then hoped to be discharged.

Lesley handed her the chocolates, and checked the clock on the wall. She had been chatting with Lynne for about an hour, and she knew she needed to get over to see how Don was. Lynne explained she was more than happy waiting for the consultant, and munching on her chocolates. Lesley was amazed at the picture of serenity her friend's mother was. Taking a deep breath, Lesley set off for Don's ward.

The maze of corridors seemed never ending, and Lesley could feel her feet beginning to ache, wishing she had been sensible enough to own a pair of trainers, never mind wear them. Wedges really weren't the footwear of choice for this type of trekking. She noticed her reflection in the large windows lining the corridors, and she could see she was already beginning to resemble someone who had undergone a strenuous session at the gym – something Lesley had never any inclination of doing – not someone visiting friends in hospital. She quickened her pace, and by the time she had reached Don's ward her hair was sticking to her head, resembling a blonde crash helmet. With Walnut Whips at the ready, and a quick pat down with her sleeve Lesley prepared to open the door to Don's room. She didn't know what to expect, and hoped she was prepared for anything.

Don was sitting on his bed, enjoying what looked like a fabulous Full English breakfast, beaming at her and professing to be enjoying every mouthful of his meal. Lesley was amazed, Don looked as bright and impeccably turned out as his wife. He too was waiting to be seen by his doctor, and then he hoped to be given the all-clear to go home. Lesley remembered she had Walnut Whips for Don and held out the now warm package. "Oooh! I haven't had these for years; I love them.' He beamed.

Lesley could feel her face reddening all the more, thanks to the combined efforts of physical exertion and the high temperature of the hospital. After sitting and chatting for a while, Lesley left Don and made her way back to Lynn. Bottled water purchased, she glugged down half its contents, stretched a little, smiling to herself as the theme tune to 'Chariots of Fire' played in her head, as she headed for the other ward. Physically panting, as Lesley reached for the handle of Lynne's room she tried desperately to smooth and style her now truly wayward hair and straighten her appearance a little.

'Darling, you look positively exhausted.' Professed Lynn, a concerned look on her face.

'No, no, I'm fine, honest.' Laughed Lesley, not admitting she was in fact completely exhausted, frazzled, and disastrously dishevelled. Lynne looking her usual fabulous self, only serving to accentuate Lesley's own bedraggled appearance. Lesley shared Lynne's delight at being told she could be discharged; just waiting for the correct paperwork so they would be able to leave.

Lesley, after catching her breath, set off once again to tell Don the good news; she surprised herself, quickly getting into her stride, and thought she might have even shaved a bit off her time as she let herself once more into Don's room. Don was delighted with the news about his wife, as was Lesley when he too confirmed he was almost ready to leave, and that he was also fine to drive himself home. After checking Don had everything ready, and arrangements made to meet him back at home, Lesley started on her way back to Lynne's room.

Doctors and nursing staff alike were now used to the sight of the blonde haired lady in the questionable footwear zipping along the busy corridors, nodding to her as she passed. 'Last time I think.' She called out to the orderly she had passed twice already throughout the day, and who had suggested she may actually want to consider getting a job at the hospital.

By the time Lesley reached Lynne her paperwork had been signed, and she already had everything packed away. Lesley slowly, and very carefully, escorted Lynne to her car and was grateful to at last be able to sit and take a very sedate drive home, sound in the knowledge that loved ones were well and back on the mend, as she gently massaged her calves before turning the key in the ignition.

Good For A Grin
YOU'LL NEVER WALK ALONE

Mike was a member of Cambridge United's supporters club. He would stand and watch with the same group of friends every Saturday, he loved the camaraderie as much as the football. When he finally decided to tell his group of mates one Saturday afternoon that he had prostaate cancer, the group fell silent.

It was obvious nobody knew what to say, until one of them finally spoke up. "It is the most common cancer for men. Many have different treatments and outcomes differ." He ended with, "I'm sure you'll be alright, Mike." Mike was thankful for the statement as, he suspected, were the rest of the group. The heavy silence was broken. It was appreciated by all.

Mike had his surgery.

Cambridge United were playing at home. It was the first game Mike had missed due to prostate cancer. At 3pm there came a text. It read: "At the slightest sign of cancer you are not here. What's the matter with you?" Mike would have laughed out loud if he wasn't still suffering from the after-effects of the operation. He certainly felt good at having received the text and mused how odd it was that someone berating you can have such a great effect and lift your spirits.

He replied with a text saying he was at home, nice and warm, being made lots of cups of tea, eating biscuits and listening to the commentary on the radio, in the hope of making them jealous. It didn't work.

Might Make You Smile
ON THE RUN

Clare had made a promise to herself; if she was well she would continue to run. She found running made her feel free and provided a great sense of well-being, as well as keeping her fit. Feeling the blood coursing through her, releasing the feel-good endorphins, and making her feel stronger and more capable of dealing with whatever life threw her way. When she was diagnosed with cancer, Clare knew so long as she was fit and strong enough; she would try and continue to run. During the treatments Clare ran as often as she was able, not always as far as she had in the past, but she viewed a run was a run, regardless of distance.

It was a good day, Clare was feeling well and looking forward to the run. With time to herself at last, she set out on the cold, bright morning. The air was crisp, and she felt it's chill against her skin. Breathing deeply and allowing the air to fill her lungs, she felt good, she felt alive.

Clare found the pounding of her feet against the pavement and uneven grassland therapeutic. Her heart felt lighter, and as she broke into her stride, the weight that seemed to nestle on her shoulders lifted. Coming around her last full circuit, she saw the lights of the local bakers cast a glow across the pavement in front of her. Quickly she ducked into the doorway, the bell over the door ringing as she stepped into the glowing interior. The warmth from within hit Clare in the face with a warm pow! In the very same moment Clare felt her nose twitch dramatically, and then with no warning, she felt a warm gush and was aware of a splashing sound on the tiled floor. It was a full minute before she saw there had been numerous splashes onto the tiled floor.

Clare realised the splashing had emanated from her. Simultaneously a handkerchief was handed to her by the lady behind the counter. 'I'm so sorry.' Clare laughed. As she quickly dabbed at her nose, she was engulfed in a mixture of embarrassment and unable to ignore the funny side of a full on gushing nose for all the world to see. She may well have lost her full head of hair, but she had not even comprehended nasal hair. She didn't even recall it being mentioned, but then she hadn't always fully listened to the dozens of possible side effects from her cancer treatment.

With a tissue held firmly to her nose, she collected the loaf she had ordered, tucked it under her arm, and headed back out into the cool air. Jogging back home Clare developed a stitch, she couldn't help but laugh at how she must have looked; laughing and jogging didn't really mix. Who knew nasal hair was so important?

Good For A Grin
SHAVE?... NOT SHAVE?

Hair loss. Not just top-of-the-head hair loss – all-over hair loss.

Now, for a man this often means goodbye razor, shaving and all the accoutrements and paraphernalia that go along with this. Depending on whether you are a man who has to shave once a day regardless, or every few days, there is a little novelty to realising you don't have to spend that time carrying out the tedious task.

If, however, you are a bearded man, the effect can be very disconcerting, even more shocking than losing the hair on your head. Thought-provoking stuff, discovering you may have an extra chin, or worse, chins that you have never had to encounter before.

As for silky-smooth legs? Not generally a priority for the male population, and a little startling when first noticed, but if you are a competitive bodybuilder, professional cyclist or just plain 'a little out there', this look may work for you. Just saying, is all.

What is undeniable is that these little day-to-day occurrences make you really appreciate things even more when they start returning to normal. The five o'clock shadow makes an appearance – cause for celebration, break out the champers! Or at least a brewski.

If you had a beard, it slowly but surely returns, and you will love it all the more. You will want to spend a little extra on that trim or try new hairstyles, guaranteed.

The household fight for the last razor will have more meaning and, though not always admitted to, appreciated tenfold.

Might Make You Smile
LOVE YOU, MUM

Sadie was someone who had seen a bit in her lifetime; having been involved in show business for decades, even having a recording career in the 1980's. All this meant she had come across a myriad of personalities. Sadie was more than capable of dealing with those who crossed her path; she liked to say she had "a look", a withering glare than sent many a combatant back from whence they came.

In dealing with her cancer, Sadie was equally defiant. She held the view that it was her cancer, and she would take it on any way she chose. This was Sadie's thinking from the offset. If she chose to deal with it with humour, however dark, that was how it was going to be, no questions asked.

Sadie was due for another bout of treatment, and whilst she was preparing for her second dose a nurse asked if it would be possible to tattoo two dots on her chest? This meant that whenever she came for subsequent treatments the dots would be aligned, and no further markings or adjustments would need to be made. The equipment could be aligned correctly on every occasion, and this would save an awful lot of time all round.

All this was explained in great detail to Sadie, who found the whole concept amusing, and her mind was already working mischievously. Sadie smiled, and then said 'You can do this of course, but can I have "I Love You Mum" tattooed instead?' The staff were momentarily speechless, and the room broke out into raucous laughter.

One nurse looked on disapprovingly, visibly tutting at the hilarity before her. Sadie caught the look on the nurse's face and flashed "the look", full beam, straight at her. Sadie and the nurse never crossed paths again, she did, however, have only the dots tattooed.

Good For A Grin
QUESTIONING PROFESSOR HAWKING

Peter had been at sea from the age of fifteen; the ocean was his calling. After many decades of circumnavigating the globe, aboard everything from tankers to cruise liners, he and his family had settled in Essex – Mersea Island to be exact.

Peter had married a beautiful South African nurse and they had two children; they were all used to sunnier climes and Mersea came as a bit of a shock. Although originally from Plaistow, Peter had loved everything about South Africa. The family had moved back to England in 1986 when he had the job of outfitting a cruise ship called The Astor from top to bottom.

It was only when he was diagnosed with a very rare form of cancer and had to undergo a dramatic and life-changing operation – a radical amputation – that he slowed down. During his hospitalisation he had many visitors, one of his regulars being his nephew Del. Del was renowned for his mischievous antics, and had brought a smile more than once to his uncle's face throughout the cancer treatment and rehabilitation.

Peter was an avid reader, a highly intelligent man, and was working his way through two of Professor Stephen Hawking's books. On one occasion Del's visit coincided with a particularly down day for Peter; Del could see he was going to have to pull out all the stops to help his uncle. After he messed around with the copious amounts of rubber gloves that were to hand in Peter's room – to the exasperation of the nurses – Peter's mood had lifted a little.

When Peter was taken for therapy, Del found the two books on his uncle's bedside cabinet. Del knew Peter would be some time and had an idea for something to leave his uncle when he returned.

Del returned the following day; he could hear his uncle before even seeing him. Peter was sitting up in bed, voicing his outrage at what he was reading. Del was privileged enough to be greeted by a barrage of expletives, as Peter explained how ridiculous he found Hawking's writing and findings. He was in the middle of ranting about how the world-renowned theoretical physicist couldn't write a book for toffee, and how he continually contradicted himself, and was frankly a fool.

It was as Peter saw his nephew's reaction that he realised something was afoot. "Go on, what did you do?" Del reached into the bedside cabinet. Realisation spread across Peter's face. "You swapped the books around, didn't you?" There followed another tirade of unprintable words – the bookmark had been placed on the same page but in the second book.

As Del left Peter's bedside that day and made his way down the corridor, he was pleased with the fact that his uncle could still be heard laughing, albeit punctuated with the occasional curse.

Might Make You Smile
AND THE AWARD GOES TO...

The boys had finally agreed to haircuts; having spent all summer looking like a cross between seven-year-old hippies or Old English Sheepdogs, with eyes close to being obscured by blonde wavy locks.

Nancy had asked her offspring to go and get haircuts. Haircuts were deemed a 'blue job' in her household. Having twin boys and one girl it was decided, with as near as possible democracy, with there being two females and three males, that there were now 'blue jobs' and 'pink jobs', especially as the children were growing up.

When Nancy had her cancer treatment explained to her she came very quickly to some decisions; her shoulder length, golden-streaked hair would have to go. She didn't think she could stand watching it fall out and, although there was no guarantee it would happen, she didn't want any further variable on top of dealing with the actual cancer.

Nancy had broached the subject with her family. Tabitha, being five, was easier to persuade a haircut was in order than the boys, Ben and Luke. It amazed Nancy how much her sons held on to her appearance. She wondered, if they perhaps saw no change, then there was nothing wrong; a sort of childlike 'head in the sand' approach. Nancy had been honest with her children about her illness, but in a very basic manner. They didn't need to know the specifics, but they did need to know mummy wasn't her normal self, and a few changes would need to be made.

Nancy's husband was a man who didn't care if his wife had long hair, short hair, or no hair at all. He had long ago shown that his love for his wife had little to do with her appearance. He had already joked with her about sporting a Sigourney Weaver from 'Aliens' look, and wasn't in the least bit surprised when Nancy told him that was exactly what she was going to do; she was going to have her hair shaved off in one go. The boys were outraged initially, but after Nancy and her husband had taped and stapled pictures from magazines of various film stars and celebrities sporting shorn looks they had finally calmed down.

What Nancy didn't tell them was that she intended to keep her hair in a little cloth pouch she had made for it. She planned a competition for the end of the summer holidays; as the boys hated having their own hair cut, she had allowed them to grow it over the summer, with the proviso they had good haircuts at the end of it.

At the same time as their haircuts, Nancy knew she would need to get her own done. Her treatment would have started, and she wanted her hair gone before it started to fall out on its own; she knew that would be far more distressing for all concerned than any haircut.

The haircut day came. Mike, Nancy's husband, was under strict instructions; short haircuts, but the hair from both boys was to be collected and put into ziplock bags and be brought home. Mike thought Nancy's idea was great. Nancy was having her hair shaved on the same morning, Tabitha was at her auntie's; Nancy felt this needed to be something done between her and her son's.

By lunchtime, everybody looked very different. Nancy was already home when she heard Mike's car pull up. For the first time, Nancy felt slightly nervous. She was less shocked by her own appearance than she had thought she would be, and she hoped her children would feel the same. She had deliberately changed her look to try and make her new image whole. She was sporting jeans, a black sweatshirt, and lace up boots, looking more like a shorn Lara Croft than her usual 'country casual' style.

She heard the key in the lock. 'Ta-da' Nancy jumped out into the hallway as the three members of her family came through the front door, there was a stunned silence. Nancy felt her breath catch in her throat, a big smile on her face, and executing what she hoped was her 'cool mum' pose.

'Mum, you look fantastic!' Luke squealed

'Mum, you look so cool!' Ben laughed.

The relief Nancy felt almost made her burst into tears, and she stood for a moment, stemming the tears that were in danger of spilling onto her cheeks.

'That's not all,' she laughed 'We now have a competition too.' Nancy held both their hands and walked her sons into the lounge. Mike had the two bags of hair clippings, Nancy had hers.

'Drum roll please Daddy' said Nancy, as she took the three bags and told the boys there was a special prize for the person, or persons, whose hair clipping pile was the biggest. Nancy had already doctored her pile to be the smallest. The boys by this point had completely forgotten about their mother's change of appearance, and were concentrating on the competition. The drum roll was reaching a crescendo; the results were in. The tie between the boys was agreed with a great deal of whooping and dancing, and a prize of a new game for each of them was given. Nancy's hair was never long again, but it took a few more haircuts for Ben and Luke before they realised they were not going to get a new game every time they got their hair cut.

Good For A Grin
MAN BABY

Looking back, there was a silver lining to all that had gone on. Nick was revelling in the new lease of life he had with his son, spending lots of time together doing silly things, like skipping through town. Nick couldn't have cared less, his sole focus was on his son and having fun with him. True, they did get some funny looks. Why was Gollum from Lord Of The Rings running through the town, skipping along with a child? As no police or social services were called, Nick guessed he couldn't have scared anyone too much.

Even when the chemotherapy made Nick very poorly, he never lost the ability to have fun. However, it had not been an easy journey.

At first the news had been devastating. The cloud of despair was all engulfing and the questions came thick and fast. When am I going to die, is it next week, next month, next year? What about my son? How do I tell him? These questions hit like a hammer blow.

Being a little nervous, Nick wanted to know when his chemotherapy was going to start. He thought he had the Christmas period to process the information he had been given, but there was to be another shock – he was to start his treatment six days later. Wow! The hits just kept on coming.

By December Nick was enjoying a cup of tea with his parents, having completed the first cycle of his chemotherapy. He absentmindedly stroked his beard, and a clump came off in his hand; and there was another shock when he checked his hair (he was normally bald but was currently sporting a sort of 'monk do') – yep, it had begun to fall out. Nick went home, took a razor to what was left and got rid of the lot.

After a day or so, Nick began to kinda like his new look; yes, he was rocking it. He may have likened his appearance to a fetus, a man baby, particularly when came the day he was completely hairless – yes, even down there. Strange feeling, strange look. It still made him smile when he recalled that the weirdest aspect of being completely 'body bald' was breaking wind for the very first time, fearing he had in fact experienced 'follow through', but hugely relieved to discover a fart was just a fart after all.

Not even when he resembled Fungus The Bogey Man after catching a cold, coupled with an infection towards the very end of his treatment and there being sufficient gunk emitted that the title seemed entirely apt, did he give up on what life had to offer. Nick was adamant his life was what he made of it, and he made so very much of every minute with his friends, family and fun. He also went on to marry again, inherit a second son and is loving life.

Might Make You Smile
A BIT LIKE GROOMING THE DOG

Susan knew her hair was falling out. It was almost as if whenever she lifted her fingers to her head she came away with some hair in her hands.

Both she and her husband Casey had made sure their children were as accepting as possible of Susan's changing appearance, her general wellness and the fact that mummy wasn't well, as accepting as two young boys could be anyway. They wanted them to understand that everything mummy was going through was going to get her better. Wherever possible, the children were involved with little things to do with Susan's treatment and recovery. They were only small, the youngest barely a toddler, but they would help with tidying the toys away and sorting out clothes for school; little things that helped Susan and Casey when tiredness from the treatments took its toll.

Susan made the decision to get rid of what hair she had left. Her idea was to make sure that her children suffered minimal shock, and the way she thought that would be best achieved would be for them to be involved with the process. Coming up with a competition, Susan planned to get her children to race to see who could gather the most hair from mummy's head, using their hands, running them through her hair.

Susan did wonder what the boys would make of her idea, but thankfully they loved it. The competition was set, and there was a prize for the winner.

'On your marks, get set, go!' Announced their Dad, and with one son on each side of her Susan began to feel little hands rummaging through her hair. The boys loved the feel of the soft hair, and weren't in the least bit concerned as the soft tufts of hair filled their hands.

There were two small piles of hair, one on either side of Susan on the table which steadily grew. Soon the hair was pretty much gone from Susan's head. The warm hands on Susan's head felt almost natural, her children were having fun, doing an albeit unusual task. It was a task that needed to be done, one way or another, and what better way to make an event less shocking for two small boys than to get them involved? It saved on a visit to the hairdressers to boot!

The judging began, both boys had impressive piles of hair, and they were both clearly proud of their efforts. With backs turned to the competitors, both Mum and Dad conferred in whispered tones. There was a heavy pause; the children waited silently.

"The judges have decided to call the competition a draw." Casey pronounced in his most official voice. The whoops and cheers from the children and parents alike were loud and prolonged. Both boys were then given a prize, happy and very proud.

Good For A Grin

VINDALOO... DON'T MIND IF I DO.

Steve had endured his rounds of chemo with his usual bravado. He had experienced some of the warned-about side effects but still felt he had come away fairly unscathed.

He had found chewing gum helped with the almost permanent dry mouth. If he felt ulcers beginning to form he would try a milkshake, the alkaline of the milk helped a little with the discomfort. Also, an unusual but handy tip for itchy hands and feet (having begun to wonder if he was developing athlete's foot, the toes on one foot being so itchy) was to rub Vick's Vapour Rub on his feet and even his hands for some relief (hoorah! for the internet and people's crazy cures). All these things are worth remembering and trying, he decided.

Having had only occasional nausea, he found peppermint tea helped alleviate the symptoms a little. Mind you, he did wonder if it was more the disgusting taste of the tea that helped distract his mind from the feeling of nausea.

About six weeks after the end of his treatment had ended, Steve noticed some unusual changes in himself. He had always been a cider drinker, but now he preferred bitter, and he had always been someone who couldn't really handle spicy food. A chicken korma to him was as much of a spicy kick as he could endure. His preference with food had always been creamy sauces, mild cheeses and subtle flavours.

It was only when he was enjoying a night out with the lads, treatment over and feeling on top of the world, did Steve discover his tastes had changed, not just a little bit but dramatically. It was the first real night out he had had in an age. The treatment had taken a little over six months in total, and this, coupled with six weeks of recovery, meant it was a while before he felt he was himself again. The evening was planned by Steve's mates and had been in the diary for some time. He was not the 'designated driver', so Steve had decided he was going to enjoy it. When (after a few beers to start with) the waitress came to take the group's food order, they decided, among other dishes, they would partake in the 'Challenge Chicken Wings' – chicken wings in a buffalo sauce made with Scotch Bonnet chilli peppers.

It was to be a shared challenge, and the idea was that the first person to eat most of the wings, sauce and everything that came with the dish was to be the winner. The group, Steve included, were all laughing at his ability, or the lack of it, to eat spicy food, and it was generally agreed that he would come last. But it would be a laugh to see who exactly would win.

The bets were in and a little wager was placed by each man. The Challenge Wings arrived. It was agreed nobody would eat their main course until the challenge had been completed. The 'dumbing down' of taste buds was not allowed with either food or drink. The challenge was on.

First to go was Mick, the largest member of the group. In his own eyes, a world-renowned 'hot chilli' eater. The first molten mouthful went down easily. The same was said for each member of the rest of the group. Then it was Steve's turn. There was much heckling and jostling as he prepared to down the forkfull. The general consensus was this would be his first and last mouthful.

The forkful of fiery spice went down easily. No one was more surprised than Steve himself. There was the odd accusation that perhaps he had consumed contraband in the form of cough sweets or something similar to numb his mouth. Round two was the same. By round three some of the group had conceded defeat and by round four there were only three contestants left in the running, Steve being one of them.

Steve couldn't believe it, not only did he find the heat and spiciness of the dish palatable, but he was actually really enjoying every mouthful – another first. In the next round the other two challengers conceded, and just to prove he really was enjoying his newfound tastes, he finished off the dish completely.

"Next time fellas, whose up for a vindaloo?" Steve laughed.

Chemotherapy hadn't just made him well again it had resulted in a whole different and new side to himself. Steve was loving it, although he wasn't however sure how much his girlfriend would appreciate his breath later.

Might Make You Smile
MAY THE FORCE BE WITH YOU

Tana received the confirmation of her breast cancer via a phone call, while out collecting holiday money with her husband. It was a surreal moment with life buzzing around her, people shopping, talking on mobile phones. Life was carrying on and yet hers, in contrast, felt like it had ground to a halt; all time had stood still. Tana was a practical woman who was always mindful of those around her, especially loved ones.

The phone call had been taken as Tana was busy, and it was only when her and her husband were walking home that she broke the news to him in her usual stoic fashion. They walked and talked about all the possible outcomes of the conversation Tana had just had over the phone. Tana made light of the situation, and declared her boobs were a bit under the weather. She was adamant her condition would not be talked of in hushed tones, or only behind closed doors. Both her and her husband decided that names should be given for her boobs, making talking about them easier; she loved the fun aspect of the conversation. Her husband came up with a few that were not exactly what she had in mind. Eventually, they settled on Milly and Boo. Tana felt it would be easier to say she was having a problem with Milly or Boo. These then evolved into Mills and Boon; what could be easier than saying she was having a 'Mills and Boon' moment?

The hard part, as is often the case, was telling the rest of the family. They were a close family, despite living all over the world, and kept in contact regularly. Once the family was told, there was the decision to set up a WhatsApp group so they could all keep up to date with developments. What Tana wasn't aware of was there was a second group created, so the family were able to air their feelings or fears without Tana being aware of them. This meant that they gave their best positivity and good vibes to Tana, and kept any worries to themselves. Tana got nothing but the upbeat, positive, and healing conversations. The family could have their private meltdowns, but they were never shown or expressed to Tana; the WhatsApp groups worked perfectly. All were given 'Star Wars' character names, Tana being a massive Star Wars fan, and of course she was Princess Leia, abbreviated to PL.

After vast amounts of research, talking to others and asking countless questions, Tana decided to have surgery. The surgery went well, and her recovery was commented on as remarkable. As was her style, Tana found an upside to the major surgery she had undertaken; it came with a free tummy tuck! Bonus!

Good For A Grin
THESE BOOTS ARE MADE FOR WALKING

Barry was a keen walker. After his prostatectomy he had wanted to indulge his passion all the more. A lust for life after the drama of the diagnosis of prostate cancer, surgery and the subsequent after-effects made him appreciate even more what life has to offer. He felt privileged to have been given another chance, another bite at the cherry.

As time wore on and he was able to take up more walking trips and excursions, Barry began to feel that incontinence during long walks was becoming a real problem.

It was suggested that the use of an external catheter could be the way forward. In order to go ahead with this, Barry had to be 'fitted' for it. The fitting involved two nurses, measuring both length and girth of his penis. Interesting, to say the least. Then came the actual fitting, one of the nurses holding the penis while the other nurse rolled the condom-type device on. So that the device would stay in place, the penis had to be held for a while so that the gel on the inside of the 'condom' bonded with the penis.

It would be fair to say that there was a time where such a tableau could have been considered almost dream-like. There may also have been a time when Barry (in fact, probably almost any male on the planet for that matter) would be grateful to be so accosted by two females, nurses at that!

It was, however, a one time only affair, and after the fitting had been demonstrated and Barry was clear on the instructions for performing the task himself, it became time for removing the catheter, or 'Conveen'. This was not such a 'pleasurable' experience. In fact, it was excruciatingly painful. Consider, if you will, a plaster being ripped off your most sensitive region. In Barry's opinion however, what was worse was that he had an afternoon appointment – his bladder did not fare so well in the afternoon and so he was somewhat desperate for the toilet by the time the nurses had finished. Perhaps not his finest moment, he considered.

However, Barry found the gains from using the 'Conveen' or external catheter have allowed his life to continue with great walking adventures, and he is a firm supporter of the device. So, if like Barry you enjoy outdoor activities or just an active lifestyle, this may be the way forward for you.

Might Make You Smile
FOR THE CAMERA

Irene had decided she would go and visit the local ladies support group, Brafternoon. She had been toying with the idea for a while and had decided today was the day. It took some courage, but she was sure when she got there and met other ladies, met the people she had heard so much about, she would be fine. Having had breast cancer, she wanted to connect with others, share in some of the positivity she had been told emanated from the group, its attendees, and organisers.

The hotel was beautiful, the day bright and sunny. Irene could hear the laughter and chatter as she approached the already open doors of the Garden Room where the group held their sessions.

With the sun streaming in, and the friendly vibe emanating from the room, Irene stepped inside. In a moment Irene was greeted with open arms and a sea of smiling faces, greetings were coming left and right. The room seemed to shine from within with happiness and positivity. Irene was asked to sign in, and was then shown to a table where there was tea, coffee, and biscuits; the place felt more like a ladies lunch party than a support group. Once Irene had got herself a drink she was introduced to a few of the other ladies, and then the organiser, Anita, asked if she wouldn't mind having a photograph taken for publicity purposes.

Irene was stumped for a moment. Pointing to her chest she replied 'What, a picture of these?' she smiled gesturing to her breasts. The roar of laughter was deafening. 'Your face, your face,' laughed the photographer rolling her eyes while trying to stop laughing as she focused the lens.

A great entrance to a great afternoon and a great day.

Good For A Grin
DRIER IF I HAD BEEN IN A CAR WASH

Dan had never been a man to sport a buzzcut. Short back and sides? Definitely. A long, shaggy Bon Jovi look? Not that he would ever admit to or provide evidence of, no. However, what Dan was completely unaware of and has a new-found respect for is those of us who are cranially hair-free, by whatever means. And if it's through choice, you are a far braver person for sure.

Chemotherapy had seen to it that Dan's hair was going, and he had to do something about it. Being honest, it was more a case of realising that the little clumps that were being deposited on the pillow, closely followed by more in the shower, meant the decision to go the whole hog and be rid of what was left was made. No comb-over attempts to be made here.

Stepping out of the barbers he was overcome by two emotions. The first was self-consciousness on a grand scale. Was everyone looking at him now he was effectively bald? Obviously, no, no they were not. Nobody who walked past turned and stared, nor was he paid any further attention than he might have been on any other occasion. The second emotion was a degree of vulnerability; even short hair can be seen as something to hide behind, it is part of our persona. There is also the feeling of not being quite as protected from the elements as before.

Anyway, fighting these two emotions and putting his best efforts into giving off an air of confidence – yes, I chose to do this – he made his way down the busy street.

Having only gone a few shop fronts down, he felt the first 'plop'. The sky darkened quickly and within seconds there was a downpour. Dan had no idea of the consequences of torrential rain and a bonce that was now as smooth as a baby's bottom. There is zero absorption other than your clothes. Very quickly, Dan realised why a hat, be it a flat cap, baseball, beanie – it matters not – is often sported by those with no hair in inclement weather.

He did begin to wonder whether there had ever been a case of drowning by downpour. If not, he thought, I may well be the first. Dan actually felt as if he were standing in a carwash, hardly able to catch his breath. He had never been so soaked, so quickly. The water fell like a sheet over his face, straight down his neck and in his ears. Yes, ears can get waterlogged in rain. The collar of his coat did nothing other than fill like a sponge, and then, when it had reached capacity, water steadily seeped down his neck, chest and back.

The only thing that might have helped would have been a squeegee. Soaked to the bone, in a very literal sense, in a matter of minutes.

From that day Dan always kept a hat of some sort in his coats, his car, the wife's car and just about any place there was room to stuff one. After the first experience he did consider keeping a set of nose clips handy too.

Might Make You Smile
WIND, WHAT WIND?

Michelle had gone through so much treatment, and so many procedures, that she almost felt as though there was nothing else she could have.

Alas, further treatment was required, and Michelle, with renewed stoicism, accepted the decision. Unfortunately, her veins were not particularly compliant, and the medical staff were having a devils-own job of getting a vein to comply and accept the needle. After what seemed like a lifetime, it was decided there may be an accepting vein found in her arm, and the needle was to be placed there. Once the needle was finally placed, the nurse left the room.

Michelle sat with nothing but her own thoughts, while her treatment took place. Her arm began to swell. A million thoughts ran through Michelle's head as she tried to will the arm to stop swelling, wondering if this was what was supposed to happen? She had been told to alert anyone if she began to feel unwell, or noticed anything unusual. Not knowing if the swelling was unusual or not, and acknowledging she didn't feel any different, she was questioning herself constantly.

A nurse popped her head round the door. 'Are you ok?', 'Have you had wind?' Michelle was taken aback. 'No, I don't think so? Should I have? I don't feel gassy, should I burp? What should I do if I do? What does it mean if I have wind?' As Michelle worriedly fired the questions out she knew she was beginning to sound a little hysterical, but was genuinely concerned as to what she should and shouldn't be experiencing.

The nurse looked at her with a quizzical expression, one eyebrow raised. She paused for a moment and cleared her throat 'No, have you had Wyn, our little South African nurse tend to you at all?' The nurse pointedly replied, still looking sceptically at Michelle.

Michelle felt her whole body relax, and she burst out laughing. The nurse smiled at her, but it was obvious to Michelle the whole situation was far funnier to her than to the nurse, even after she was able to explain the joke.

Good For A Grin
UNCLE FESTER

Sid had felt lousy for a long time. Not only due to lethargy and a lack of appetite, but also from being unable to sleep at night, plus significant weight loss. All of this, accompanied by persistent nagging from his wife, finally saw him wind up at the doctors surgery.

That day he received the news he was dreading: he had non-Hodgkin's lymphoma. What followed next in the conversation was a complete blur and Sid was totally unable to recollect anything further.

Within two weeks he had a chemotherapy treatment plan in place. After scan upon scan he was told he had a very good chance of a complete recovery. Prednisolone was prescribed and his life took on a new dimension.

Sid marvelled at just how quickly he and his family adapted to the new way of life – driving to appointments, people organising their days around his needs. Sid felt truly blessed to have such amazing family and friends around him.

The effects from his treatment took hold quite quickly. He gained weight, lost all his hair, but his grandchildren took it all in their stride. In some respects more so than the adult members of the family.

It was almost winter time, Halloween was a couple of days away and the grandchildren were getting their costumes ready. Trick or treating was the order of the day, well, evening.

Sid had an idea. He found a huge woollen coat in a local charity shop. It was enormous, even for his now increased size. With dark circles courtesy of eyeshadow around his eyes, and his completely bald head, he made the perfect Uncle Fester from The Addams Family.

The grandchildren were delighted when Grandad joined them for the whole evening trick or treating. They beamed with pride when their friends said: "Your Grandad is so cool! His costume is ace." The trick-or-treat booty for that year was record breaking. Sid had a blast and was happy to share the treasure.

Watching his grandchildren chomping their way through the sweet treats, he had to smile at the irony that having cancer had given him the perfect Halloween costume and a permanent, unique memory of precious, fun times spent with his grandchildren.

As the saying goes, every cloud… has a silver lining.

Might Make You Smile
WHITE AS A GHOST

Elsie and her younger roommate Cathleen had the same cancer, and were undergoing similar treatments. The ladies were laying in their respective beds, bemoaning as to their unkempt appearances. They had both wanted to have their hair washed, but they couldn't, and it was beginning to get them down.

Neither woman had any 'dry shampoo', which they were sure would help them feel better; a little more groomed if nothing else. One of the nurses had heard their complaints and had suggested talcum powder as an alternative. Initially, Cathleen and Elsie had laughed at the suggestion, but after a moment's contemplation Elsie decided she would give it a go.

Sitting on the edge of her bed, still laughing at the suggestion but desperate to make some improvement in her appearance, she carefully twisted the top of her talcum powder bottle. The pleasant aroma wafted up, and Elsie joked that if nothing else, her hair would smell nice.

Listening to the nurse's instructions, she had intended to lightly sprinkle the top of her head and then comb through the powder evenly. This, the nurse assured her, would leave her hair smelling fresh, looking clean, and easier to style; she would feel like a new woman. Cathleen watched her friend getting prepared, and she decided she would give it a go as well.

Unfortunately, what actually happened next was not quite what they expected. As soon as Elsie tipped the powder bottle upside down the top came off completely, and the entire contents was deposited on top of her head, shoulders and face. Without saying a word she turned to Cathleen, who was laughing uncontrollably, and unable to help in any way. Elsie was completely white, her eyes blinking through her ghost-like face. She couldn't help but laugh at herself, as the powder fell in great fragrant clouds around her with every movement. 'You look like a ghost.' Cathleen was finally able to say, her side aching from all the laughter. It was at that exact moment that the buzzer rang, indicating visiting time had just begun. Both Elsie and Cathleen were still having fits of giggles, Elsie still white but beautifully fragrant as the first visitors of the day arrived.

Good For A Grin
EDITED NEWS

Peter was a man, much like any other man – he tended not to fuss. He was a person who was inclined to play things down and was in most cases a calm and measured individual.

This actually translates to: doesn't really say anything when something is wrong, until it is almost too late; puts off something as not being particularly important but actually is; a tendency to brush things aside.

These traits are borne out of protection and love for those closest to him, although sometimes sprinkled with a large dose of denial.

When Peter discovered he had cancer he dealt with it in his usual manner. It was nothing really, everything will be fine. This was by no means a bad outlook, and better than being the other way for sure, but it can be a little confusing for loved ones, friends and family.

Peter's daughter was keen for updates on her father's treatment and how he was feeling/coping. She soon learnt that she had to adopt a two-pronged approach. She would message her dad directly and he would reply with plenty of upbeat, positive and often hilarious renditions of the day's activities, events and how he was feeling. This she would take huge comfort from as she knew that he was being 'Dad', which in itself was a great sign.

She would then message her step-mother and get the more realistic take on events.

If Peter was suffering a little from niggly aches and pains and wasn't quite as chipper as on previous occasions, she took this to mean that he was actually feeling pretty awful, wasn't getting out of bed until late, and was feeling down and a bit bad tempered. As he was perfectly entitled to feel. It was his language and she understood it completely.

This system allowed her dad to deal with his illness his way, protect his loved ones and keep things the way he wanted them – and his wife was able to provide a true account of her husband's state of health.

Dad did the edited version, step-mum did the warts-and-all.

The family was therefore both well informed and handling Peter's cancer 'their' way. There is only one rule when dealing with cancer: "There are no rules."

Might Make You Smile
OPPOSITE ENDS

Myer, through her experiences as an oncology nurse, found there were two subjects that were sometimes taboo. One was sex, and the other was poo.

These two topics often had folks divided. There were some patients, who often referred to themselves as 'frequent flyers', that had suffered more than one run-in with cancer. These were seasoned patients who had been there, seen it, done it, and got the T-shirt. They were happy to drop their underwear in a heartbeat to show off a newly healing radiotherapy site, or give a full and frank account of their findings with their latest stool sample, and how it came to be. As for sex, there would often be red faces all around as they divulged details of their sex lives. One man even commenting on just how unaffected his libido was, even though he was undergoing a gruelling chemotherapy regime, much to the utter embarrassment of his wife sat next to him.

The other end of the spectrum was often the newly diagnosed who, on top of being given sometimes devastating, certainly life changing news, then had to start revealing and recording the ins and outs of the most personal and private parts of their lives. Myer was always amazed how, in the end, everything was covered; the embarrassment was put aside, all matters were dealt with, even with a smile or two.

As a nurse, all cancers, treatments, and symptoms were approached with a caring and open mind, and always with an adaptability to the person's own mood. Throughout all her dealings,

Myer always felt that her patients, be they young or old, were always looking for the next reason to laugh or make someone in the room smile. As a nurse, Myer felt it was her job to take her patients lead, and always walk into every unit, every day, with a smile for every patient.

Good For A Grin
AHH, GOT A NEW FRIEND?

Day 1 Cycle 1

Dan arrived at Marsden Hospital in Sutton and was shown to Kennaway Ward. Blood tests, urine tests and having a canula installed was the order of the day.

Dan was given the daily menu to peruse, featuring breakfast, lunch and dinner with as much tea, coffee and biscuits on demand, much to wife Nat's amusement – she couldn't help but remark that the ward was more like a spa. All this as the day's sun shone through the large windows.

It was on the ward that Dan was introduced to Gethyn, a rugby lad (that is a guaranteed instant rapport) who played locally until he moved back to Wales. Gethyn had undergone the same surgery and was about to embark on the same BEP3 treatment with the same cycle dates. Firm 'chemo friends' status was established and posted, much to the amusement of Dan's 'Poppy Boys' (a group of friends who are the husbands of the mum's group at the local boys' school) and his rugby mates.

With this new 'friend' status being broadcasted, there then followed a deluge of 'friends' memes from The Inbetweeners. Gotta love your mates. Bastards.

Might Make You Smile
HELLO LITTLE OLD LADY

Margaret was visiting her sons for the weekend. She loved spending time with her family and getting involved with their everyday lives. With her cancer treatments taking up so much time and effort it was good to be in the thick of normal family life, with its everyday ups and downs. Her chemotherapy had taken its toll, and she had lost all of her hair. She was sitting at the dressing table, trying to work out how to make herself feel and look vaguely human again, when her six-yead-old granddaughter came into the room and sat beside her.

Margaret had a scarf draped over her head, and her granddaughter Lola sat beside her, looking at her grandmother's reflection in the mirror; the two contemplated one another for a moment. Lola then cocked her head on one side and declared matter-of-factly, 'Oh, Nana, you look like a little old lady'. Margaret fell about laughing, thinking to herself, 'From the mouths of babes'. Lola was now laughing at her Nana, who was incapable of talking for laughing. Margaret marvelled at how children have the ability to be brutally honest, but never with malice; they simply tell it as they see it.

Margaret hugged her granddaughter tightly and began to wind the scarf around her head, still chuckling to herself.

Good For A Grin
CHEMO CHROME DOME

Peter was on cycle two of his chemotherapy for his cancer treatment. He was feeling very lucky and his consultants and nurses were delighted with his progress.

He had, so far, experienced no nasty side effects, no nausea, nothing. That was until he noticed his eyebrows were thinning and his hair was beginning to, as he liked to put it, 'move away' from his head. This he truly felt was a small price to pay for getting well again. Having the sort of outlook and sense of humour he had, he mused at his reflection in the mirror as he contemplated his hair, or the continuing lack of it.

Yes, he felt he had invented a new hairstyle, one he chose to call the 'Chemo Chrome Dome', an ultra-modern affair, suitable for all ages, though only the very daring may be so bold as to sport the style.

That said, it required very little styling, merely the arranging of just two hairs. This, he considered, was perfect for today's man on the go.

Might Make You Smile
LIZZIE'S DENIAL

Lizzie was a woman who had a tendency to put everyone else's feeling before her own. This was a commendable trait for sure, however, it had a habit of leading to denial on the part of Lizzie.

When Lizzie finally got herself to the doctor, after not feeling herself for some time, she was already on the way to playing down the feelings of fatigue, constant illness, and the unexplained swelling she had discovered as something to be ignored. She could well have sabotaged herself there and then, but her doctor knew Lizzie of old and sent her straight away for tests.

The tests came back showing abnormalities, again Lizzie played the whole matter down, her family behaved accordingly. Everyone went about their business as usual. When the date for her consultant's appointment arrived Lizzie even attempted to go on her own, but her husband insisted on attending, and when the news was broken that Lizzie had cancer her response was typical. Even when she was taken into a separate consulting room to be alone with the Macmillan nurse, she insisted she was fine, and that was that.

Lizzie dismissed and trivialised as much as possible; this coming from her need to protect all those around her. It was only when her treatments began that Lizzie felt, perhaps, she was doing herself a disfavour.

There was one particular occasion, as she was suffering badly with sickness, her head firmly in the toilet bowl, with the much-loved family Labrador trying to lick her feet. She was also listening to her eldest daughter lament about lost loves, and latest boyfriend crushes, not pausing for breath other than to check that her mother was in fact still listening. Her husband was standing on the other side of the bathroom door, occasionally popping his head round to tell her what he had just discovered they had ran out of, grocery-wise, and Lizzie snapped. In between bouts of retching Lizzie firmly but politely told her daughter to buck up and shut up, gave the dog its marching orders and fished the Waitrose card out of her nearby handbag and promptly threw it in the direction of her husband, inadvertently bouncing it off her husband's head; she mumbled an apology and told him to 'go fill his boots' at the supermarket.

Within minutes the house was silent, and Lizzie was feeling a little better. Lizzie was no longer in denial, and she realised she felt so much better for it. Now it was time for a quiet cup of tea and to read a magazine.

Good For A Grin
POOL TABLE, COLOURFUL DÉCOR, XBOX... IS THIS THE HOSPITAL ARMS?

The last hurdle, the last bout of treatment, but there was no room at the inn!

Yes, the treatment was scheduled, but alas there was no bed on the usual ward. What to do? Nick was the youngest male on the ward he normally resided in, and fortunately there was an alternative. Seeing an opportunity for a little bartering, he asked if it was possible to have a room of his own. The nursing staff said they would see what they could do.

Not too long after he was asked to follow the nurse who was overseeing his treatment. Had he pushed his luck, was he about to be confined to a pipe-and-vent-filled basement, the clanging and hissing of the hospital bowels his only comfort and companion?

As they made their way through the corridors, it certainly didn't feel like he was heading to the murky depths of the building.

Nick was surprised – he did get his own room but it had four beds in it; but it mattered not, he was delighted. He did, however, note the colourful walls, a pool table and games console. The whole place looked more like a pub than a hospital ward.

Regardless, it was no problem, he was just pleased to be getting his treatment and in such amenable surroundings. It was in fact a children's ward. As it turned out this was no bad thing, in fact it was great! Playing pool and Xbox all day was most relaxing, and the kids were fantastic. Nick felt at home and loved the company of so many children; they were all so strong, going through the same thing as Nick, but never lost the ability to have fun and muck around. He truly felt it was a great way to finish his last round of treatment.

Might Make You Smile
HOW'S YOUR EARS?

Michelle had undergone a full hysterectomy, and was recovering in hospital. She was trying to get herself in as comfortable position as was possible under the circumstances, when a flustered consultant entered her room. He introduced himself; Michelle hadn't seen this particular consultant before, but during her treatments she had seen so many different people that it came as no surprise to meet someone new. With all the doctors and nurses coming and going in the busy ward, this was no surprise.

Bending toward Michelle, the consultant asked 'How are your ears?' Michelle was somewhat taken aback, wondering if there was a side effect that she was unaware of from the surgery. She had paid no attention to her hearing after the operation, so now that her attention was drawn to them she paused for a moment. No, her hearing was fine. 'And what about your nose?' The consultant asked. It was at this point that Michelle and her husband looked at each other questioningly. Again, Michelle's attention was drawn to her nose, a little runny maybe, but nothing untoward she decided.

The consultant then went on to examine her head area, moving her head from one side to the other, 'Well, this is very odd.' He muttered. Michelle began to panic slightly. The consultant then asked her to open her mouth, and he peered down her throat. Michelle heaved herself up straight as best she could, and opened her mouth as wide as possible. The consultant sounded exasperated and asked 'whatever is the matter with you?' Michelle explained that she was having difficulty moving due to the drains she had been fitted with after her Hysterectomy operation. "Op? Op? I'm the ear, nose, and throat specialist, not a gynaecologist. Who are you?' He asked, baffled and exasperated.

Needless to say, the consultant had gone into the wrong room, to see the wrong patient, about the wrong procedure. Michelle couldn't help but see the funny side of it all, and was pleased to know her ears were fine.

Brafternoon

WWW.BRAFTERNOON.CO.UK

Brafternoon is a not for profit group, whose sole aim is to provide a positive social experience, making a difference for ladies who have been affected by cancer.

With a wonderful setting and a great bunch of women, it has been succinctly said, that whilst 'having Cancer is a club that no one wants to be in'; 'Brafternoon is one club that everyone wants to be in!'

It offers a rare opportunity to spend time with ladies who really do understand; discussing a wide range of issues, swapping experiences and sharing activities - ultimately sharing one another's journey.

It's not all about Cancer; it's about giving women some 'me time' and an opportunity to leave everything else at the door for an afternoon.

GET YOUR BLOGGING ON!

Something that helped me massively when writing this book was the fact that some fellas had decided the way forward was to blog their journey with their cancer.

Each person had their own reason for blogging, providing a 'warts-and-all' account of every stage. It serves as a reminder to them, how far they have come and how they felt at the time, but it also provides 'real' information, removes taboos and raises awareness.

Printed in Great Britain
by Amazon